Dear Tracy
I hope this help
you. Much love
Aunt Linda
8-16-2017

Heal the Brain, Heal the Body

Linda Gifford

BALBOA.
PRESS

A DIVISION OF HAY HOUSE

Balboa Press books may be ordered through booksellers or by contacting:

Balboa Press
A Division of Hay House
1663 Liberty Drive
Bloomington, IN 47403
www.balboapress.com
1 (877) 407-4847

Because of the dynamic nature of the Internet, any web addresses or links contained in this book may have changed since publication and may no longer be valid. The views expressed in this work are solely those of the author and do not necessarily reflect the views of the publisher, and the publisher hereby disclaims any responsibility for them.

The author of this book does not dispense medical advice or prescribe the use of any technique as a form of treatment for physical, emotional, or medical problems without the advice of a physician, either directly or indirectly. The intent of the author is only to offer information of a general nature to help you in your quest for emotional and spiritual well-being. In the event you use any of the information in this book for yourself, which is your constitutional right, the author and the publisher assume no responsibility for your actions.

Any people depicted in stock imagery provided by Thinkstock are models, and such images are being used for illustrative purposes only. Certain stock imagery © Thinkstock.

Print information available on the last page.

ISBN: 978-1-5043-7360-9 (sc)
ISBN: 978-1-5043-7362-3 (hc)
ISBN: 978-1-5043-7361-6 (e)

Library of Congress Control Number: 2017901288

Balboa Press rev. date: 01/31/2017

Contents

Introduction

As George Bernard Shaw tells it "Life isn't about finding yourself. Life is about creating yourself."

Over 50, you are a classic. Just like a classic car needs to be restored, refurbished or repaired to shine once again, we too need to do the same! Are your pipes rusted, your fenders dented, does your carburetor need to be replaced, are your tires flat or your headlights burned out, just no more get and go in your engine? You may want to keep reading!

Learn how to live this part of your life with less pain, less illness and with more balance. I am free to recreate myself in the same way laws and text books change with the times. I do this by updating my understanding. Thereby I am free to make different choices!

More and more Americans are living longer than ever before. The human life expectancy is increasing, barring unforeseen circumstances. Experts say that the Baby Boomer generation will live to be 100 years old. Although our life expectancy has increased, the quality of our lives and our health often has not. It is up to us to take responsibility for our health in the next 20, 30, 40 or 50 years that we have left. You should be looking at the age of your current doctor as well. It is very likely that you will have several doctors over the course of this part of your life. I have talked with hundreds of Americans and most of them do not want to live into their 90s, let alone past 100 years old. Studies have shown that a baby born in 2014 is expected to live to be 128 years old.

Look at your past 20 or 30 years and answer this question:

Have you ever experienced illness, disease and/or disabilities? If so, you need to change the way you have been living. This book can give you tools and examples of how you can accomplish the changes needed. I hear people say over and over again that they do not want to be dependent on family, or be taken care of in nursing homes. Most Americans want to be able to take long walks, travel, play golf, and enjoy family, and friends, no matter what their age. Americans want those extra years to be quality years. Our long lives do not mean much if we are not active and productive. The quality of our coming years will depend largely on the choices we make from now on; choices designed to stave off the aging process, and not accepting the words given to us by well meaning people. Many who say "You get that way when you get old," or "That is just part of old age!" NO, I say. DO something different for yourself, NOW!

The powerful and committed women in this book share their stories and paths they took to change their health and life. They decided where they wanted to go and the choices needed to fulfill their dreams. They are on their own adventures to age with a purpose.

The stories of these women are not based on the standards of others who put aging into the familiar clichés: "Oh, forgetfulness is just part of getting old, you are having a senior moment" or "Pain happens to old people, you can't expect life without pain."

With the entire internet, books and different suggestions of the do's and don'ts, it is hard to know what is needed to create a better life for one's self. It can seem overwhelming: I have found that people want to take control of their own aging process, in their own way, by having options. This book introduces new options.

After reading their stories, you will find the methods they used, how they changed their lives and the ways you can use them in your own life. Plus, you will find scientific research on how the brain and body connection creates healing. This book gives examples, stories, and gives results; all created for easy understanding. As I have studied, listened and watched others live a longer life, I have found that life used to seem like a timeline; but I have come to realize, life is like the weather. The only thing certain is change.

Here is a story I just love to give as an example of what is meant by a timeline.

Two young girls were having a tea party outside. They were comfortably sitting at a pint size table on chairs. Each expressed kindness to the other as they sipped pretend tea from tiny tea cups. The curious, three year old asked her beautiful friend "What is it like being five?" The five year old replied, "I can tell you for sure, it's much different than being three years old!"

As you age, keep in mind this story of the difference between being three and five years old. We used to measure our aging differences in 10 year increments. In our teens we felt like_____, in our 20's we could do _____, in our 30's we better do_____, In our 40's we are in a _____ and in our 50's we are over the _____. After the 50 threshold we must measure our aging differences in two to three year increments. Take a look at your body and your life three years ago, has it changed any? Can those three years make a huge difference in the aging process? OH YES!

This book was written for and by women, although men can benefit by what is written. The first story is mine. Following my story are four stories of women who wanted better health as well as improving their aging process. Towards the back of the book there are stories of others who have worked with me for many years. The pages in between contain the research, studies and explanations of how and why I have used this incredible information.

In chapter 17 you will find instructions on how to do the techniques and tools used in this book.

> *Life is like a series of events, and putting them together like a dot to dot puzzle in a serendipitous way.*
>
> *The definition of serendipity is, level of events that take form and finding valuable or pleasant, that are not look for.*

Chapter 1

My Story, from My Point of View

Apollinaire writes: Come to the edge he said. They said we are afraid. Come to the edge he said. They came. He pushed them and they flew"

On a dark, rainy winter night I was driving, on the freeway at a safe speed of 55 MPH when all of a sudden a large, late model Chevy was spinning across the freeway up ahead. It hit the center divider, careening into oncoming traffic. Right before my eyes I realized I had no way to avoid a collision. I was hit and the impact was so great that it felt like I had slammed into a concrete wall. My body was tossed back and forth, and from side to side, the impact hitting me with a force of a tornado. My body flung around like a rag doll. In that one second my life and my family's life changed forever.

Before I knew it, I was placed on a stretcher board with my head strapped down. "Don't move," I was told as I was rushed off to the nearest hospital. The ER was exceptionally busy due to all the accidents caused by the wet slick roads. The attendant informed me that there were no rooms available. I would have to remain in the hall, until someone could take a look at me. The noise of the ER, the lights above and every smell abusively assaulted my senses.

A policeman then came up and jostled me until I woke up. I jerked and a surge of pain shot through my head as he asked for my driver's license, and my recollection of how the accident happened. I told him how the other car was traveling ahead of me in the right lane. Suddenly it hit deep water on the roadway, spinning out of control. The other car ended up in the wrong direction hitting me head on, I, stating "it was his fault." The policeman in his professional manner announced, "Madam we can't determine who was at fault because you do not have insurance." "I do have insurance!" I screamed out with my head in pain, and sick to my stomach. I was unable to think beyond that. (It took an attorney to straighten out my insurance discrepancies and I was insured.) The policeman went up the hall to converse with a doctor. The doctor called out to a nurse, "Keep an eye on her and get someone to come and pick her up. She has no insurance and we are just too busy to keep her." I was released in my sister's care and given a preprinted patient care instruction sheet, along with a written prescription for the pain and a muscle relaxant.

Days and then weeks went by; I was still in overwhelming pain. I was unable to get my primary doctor to see me, as the hospital suggested, because he didn't treat auto accident patients. "You are no longer his patient," I was told. So what was I going to do now? The medication given to me at the hospital was running out, and the pain made it hard for me to function. By now, sheer terror had set in; all I wanted to do was sleep this pain away. However, sleep was illusive because of the pain. Time was not lessening the pain. In fact it was getting worse. My sister's chiropractor friend said, "Get her into my office, she needs care, her attorney will figure out all of the insurance discrepancies." The chiropractor's specialty was auto accidents and whiplashes. Bingo, now I was getting some care. The chiropractor explained what to expect with a whiplash. The whiplash was why I could not sleep, and why my headaches were so great even with the pain medication. The chiropractor could tell I needed additional care. Within two months after the accident, an orthopedic doctor and four dental specialists were part of my health care team, along with a new primary care physician.

There were long periods of time when I wanted to do nothing. The pain was so great at times; I wanted to give up on life. The left side of my head, shoulder, hip, knee and ankle were severely injured, along with a severe whiplash. I couldn't walk beyond 20 feet without crying out. Due to the location of the seatbelt, across my torso, I had internal injuries caused by its restraining action.

That was only part of the problem. How could I get the help I needed when every part of my body screamed out. On a scale of 1 to 10, my pain was a 10, everywhere!

Later I found out that my jaw was fractured on both sides, and my sinus cavities were shattered. Too much time had passed to do much with my jaw and sinuses, as they were already starting to improperly heal. Because of the severity of the impact to my head and face the dentists knew that, if at all possible, they had to try and save my teeth. So they were willing to try, if I gave them the okay. Was this the reason I had problems eating anything but soft food and liquids? Could this be why I had trouble forming words when trying to speak? My tongue and lips just didn't work together as I tried to form sentences, consequently others could not understand me. I would have outbursts of anger and frustration while trying to communicate with them.

I tried to take control of my life, but all I was doing was sleeping, in short intervals, or crying because the pain was so great. By now a stack of medications were sitting by my bed. As I looked at them, crying, I asked myself, "Is this going to be my life from now on?"

There were long periods of time wanting to do nothing except give up on life. Whenever the pain got to be too much, or I couldn't stand my life, I would think of my grandson. My grandson gave me special moments of joy. His curiosity of life and the magical moments we had together, inspired me. There were learning moments, mixed in with delights. I tried to play video games or work blocks alongside him but I couldn't keep up. We both got frustrated, so most of the time I just watched him play, giggle and laugh. When we watched movies together, I wanted to know when the scary scenes would be coming, so I wouldn't jerk fast and give myself a worse headache. My grandson would say "Grandma, just listen to the music, the music will tell you when it is going to get scary." I did what he told me and I learned to listen. With him, I had a playmate who taught me to take one step at a time in my journey back to some semblance of myself. This was more than what the clueless adults around me could realize. Most adults just saw me as an adult getting old.

When my semi-retired primary doctor took me as his patient,

he decided, after a thorough exam, to collaborate with my attorney. He communicated that it was imperative that I get a neurological exam and a PET scan to determine the extent of my traumatic brain injury (TBI). He knew I had problems with sensory integration: and cognitive issues. In addition, he became aware of me showing signs of my invisible wounds; panic attacks, anxiety, inability to understand or remember his simple instructions, and my irritability. My moods regularly felt as if they were falling down an elevator shaft, then as swiftly as they went down, would move swiftly upward. I could tell that my body was in crisis and not having any emotional control; I was devastated.

Eighteen months passed by, and my attorney had been able to get my insurance straightened out and some of the medical bills were getting paid.

Until the accident, I was a successful professional woman who took pride in my disciplined work, dressed with style and grace; now needed others to help me with my daily care. I not only needed help with medical care, but in my personal life and finances as well. It was almost as if someone else had to function for me. I couldn't cook for myself because I might forget and leave pots cooking on the hot stove. Others wondered if I would burn down the house. All at once, life felt utterly and grimly hopeless, without any rewards or hope for a successful end.

Being overwhelmed by grief, crying for no reason, and bursting out in anger, all became the norm. Depression settled in. I felt that life had stopped short, and I became frozen in grief and despair. My words could please, wound, enrage or disappoint others at any given moment.

Those first five years after the accident were overwhelming to everyone in my life. I still can't recall the first four years. If I'm asked about these years I have to look at my notes. Those years took a heavy toll on my relationships.

I experienced over sensitive stimuli that resulted in intensified pain from bright sunlight and car headlights, along with loud sounds. Smells of food and flowers, that once gave me pleasure, disappeared. Learning to not bend down below my waist was especially hard. If I unconsciously did, it felt like a bomb going off in my head. Sleeping in a recliner and keeping my head elevated, as well as my body still, helped somewhat with my continuous pain. No medication or therapy could do more.

My eight year old grandson remained my inspiration to get better. His smiles, laughter and his touch kept me in the present moment. I seemed to remember him the best, of anyone, in those first four years.

I would carry a notebook with me at all times, even around the house. I would write down what others would tell me, and how I felt. Confused, I needed help to navigate through my everyday life. I would write down the things that needed to be done, but I couldn't always understand my notes. There were water stains in my notebook. They were not just water stains. They were tears, and plenty of them. Diagnosed with PTSD, my writing helped me to communicate with others. Two years after the accident, I was assigned a conservator, my daughter. When my daughter took over, I found out I wasn't taking care of myself. My daughter scolded me "you need to wash your hair, when did you last brush your teeth? You are wearing the same clothes the last three days!" My daughter became the mother and I became the child. No daughter or mother should be in this situation! I was this adult trying to conduct my life as an adult, but in most areas, I acted like a child and didn't even know it.

Within months after the accident, I lost my job because I was unable to do the job I was hired to do. Long-time friends, I could remember. Someone I met and spent time with, a week earlier, I could not remember our meeting or their name. Not understanding the social gatherings I attended, I would ask why I hadn't been invited, only to see myself in the pictures that I was there. Words could not express how sad this made me feel. I felt I had lost my mind and my life. What would my grandson think of me now?

Those who knew me before the accident didn't understand this new person. Everyone tried to keep me in their lives, but it got overwhelming, as my needs were too much for them to handle being near me. One by one, they started dropping out of my life. Those people were gone. In their place was a lonely void, a great hollowness was left where something lovely and solid used to be. That's as close as I could come to naming the sensation.

Those who have known me for a long time but hadn't seen me

struggle through those really uncertain times during my recovery are still with me today. Those who met me after the accident, walking with me step by step through recovery, are still in my life, encouraging me to continue living life and helping others. Those first five years were over whelming to all. Here are some statements I was told many times as I tried to get my life back. "At your age you can't expect too much. You are just getting old and that is what happens when you get old. Old people do this and act like that. You are just having a senior moment." The statement "you are getting old" didn't settle with me then and I still will not accept today.

At first I did mostly mainstream medicine, listening to my health care professionals. Unsettling to me was their opinion that I would never be able to take care of myself. They advised, to those who were responsible for me, that I would always need assistance. Mainstream medicine did give a glimmer of hope by adding physical therapy, occupational therapy, a neurologist, massage therapy and counseling. Still, I was in constant pain and living on a cocktail of eight prescription medications, including narcotics, many being toxic with multiple side effects. I was heavily reliant on my primary doctor, orthopedist, chiropractor, dentists and counselor. After I had numerous x-rays, MRI's, CT scans, ultrasounds, EKG's, blood tests and PET scan, all of my health care professionals indicated that I would not be getting much better. The PET scan showed a Traumatic Brain Injury (TBI). The ultrasounds showed multiple internal injuries. The EKG showed the condition of my heart. The MRI's and CT scans showed injuries of the spine, knee, ankle and shoulder. The x-rays revealed the jaw, teeth and sinus cavity injuries.

Now, that I had a good idea of what my injuries were and what was in store for me the rest of my life, I needed to do something for myself. I needed to add some alternative treatments into my everyday health care. Slowly, with the assistance and advice of my chiropractor and my counselor, I added the following alternative treatments, one by one.

Holistic massage therapy, cranial sacral therapy, acupuncture, acupressure, reflexology, British sports therapy, kinesiology, colon hydrotherapy, NAET, NET, EFT, KHT therapies, Pranic Healing,

Reiki, energy work, grief work, hypnosis and Super Brain Yoga, to just name a few. Many of these healing methods I became certified in, so I can teach them to others.

Just before the fifth anniversary of the accident, it was court time. Could I handle all the depositions and court questioning? I was asked by the opposing attorney to come in and give a deposition. This continued for six sessions. He would ask the same questions each time I came in. As I answered the questions, he would tell me that I was not telling the truth. He stated that the last time I was in, I answered differently. Having a traumatic brain injury, it is not easy to answer questions about an event that happened almost five years earlier. I was trying to forget that accident and get control of my life once again. Having PTSD didn't help to try and recall that horrible night over and over again. Many days went on like this and the depositions became a stack, eight inches thick, before going to court.

Four hours was tops for me on any given day. I was never able to go more than four hours at a time. Since three or four eight hour days were needed to conduct the court hearing, my attorney wondered if I could handle it. My daughter was with me those first two days, of court, but the last days I was on my own. I took many notes throughout those days and I did make it, but don't expect me to recall the court hearing now, I can't. With the hearing behind me, it was time to move on.

Going over my notes and trying to remember; of the first five or six years, I felt confused because I could not remember. Trying to do something, I used to be able to do; it frustrated me when I could no longer do it. To see the faces of my loved ones as I struggled to talk, cook, clean and take care of myself was sad for me. I got angry when they tried to talk to me about anything that I should be doing or when they tried to correct me. I would say things like "I know how to do it or I am doing it." They knew full well, I was not. I would ask a question and my grandson would say, Grandma, you have asked that question several times and we already answered it." I would say "what was the answer?" Sometimes they would give me the answer again and sometimes, in their frustration, they wouldn't. My grandson hurt my heart whenever he would say "Grandma all we know for sure is that you don't know anything." I am sure it hurt his heart to see me like that. Many times, in my notes, I have written his statement of me not knowing, but still to this day it hurts me to read it.

Looking back to move forward!

I had all my rights taken away from me, stripped down to a mere nothing; I became nobody which left me numb. You couldn't Google me, I wasn't Googleable. I woke up one day and had a zero credit score. I didn't exist! My daughter was my overall conservator for several years, until I could safely take care of myself and safely live alone. Then a friend's husband became my financial conservator, for another five years. My essential needs, like rent, utilities, and health care, were paid by each of my conservators. I had no money to my name, except, that I was given $300.00 a month to manage myself, for gas, food, and personal needs.

At the beginning, I was told an angry frustrated personality showed up in me. Freedom was all I wanted back. Freedom to be able to take care of myself financially, cook for myself, live on my own without someone telling me to do this or that, all of the time. I wanted to be able to make good decisions for myself. I want my role as a mother and grandmother be restored to a healthy relationship.

A traumatic brain injury (TBI) can leave a terrible scar on an individual, as it did on me, shattering the lives of family and friends. Support for a person with a TBI and/or PTSD is greatly misunderstood. Each in nature can be accumulative, as well as not.

Over time I eliminated the eight prescription medications I had been living on. The brain's plasticity was evident as I started to gradually eliminate the prescription drugs from my life. I use many preventive methods in my health care. When pain arrives I used a topical pain reliever or one of the alternative techniques mentioned earlier. I no longer think of popping a pill.

After recent tests, all this work has paid off. Tests show that my body and brain are 14 years younger than my actual age. I am making future plans to live to be a 100 years old, and living a healthy active and productive life! I still have problems, but I know my limits and use routine systems to manage my life. I still only cook one pot at a time, and put important notes on my front door. They remind me to pay a bill or remind me I have a list to follow to complete my daily tasks. I use a calendar book, the size of a check book, showing a whole month at once, with one inch squares for each day. I do not put more than three things in that days square.

I am still only good for four hours at a time. Within those four hours, I schedule my personal care, household care, social engagements, along with other activities. I have learned to take care of myself and no longer need a conservator. I live independently and handle my own finances. I cook and clean, take care of my own living space. I remind myself that the challenges of day-to-day responsibilities and commitments can make anyone feel overwhelmed at times. I no longer multitask; I do one thing at a time. As a priority, in my life, I focus on simplicity to create balance. When I stay connected to the simple things, in life, I feel more relaxed. When I create simplicity, I experience more ease in my life. To this day every time I get into a car I say a prayer for protection.

What I have learned, I am teaching others. Today I say; "The old self is gone and the new self has been allowed to emerge, like a butterfly coming out of a cocoon." Make no mistake, I still have problems articulating what I want to say or write. However, you can tell I did a pretty good job writing this book and I thank all those who have helped me in this endeavor. I know I am not alone and have created a good support system around me.

I have nothing left to prove. I have been knocked down, chewed up, given up on, all the while having a body riddled with pain and headaches that were beyond comprehension. I lost my identity and means of support and told I just had to live with the outcome.

That is why I work on my brain each and every day, while protecting my brain as much as possible. I had difficulty writing about myself and my experience for this book. When my emotions would come up, while writing my story, I would freeze and unable to continue for long periods of time. I often remind myself that set backs are just warm ups for success!

I want my body and my brain to be healthy and useful. I don't want to be put out to pasture, to have grass growing up around me or me rusting out. I want to be productive, useful, and respected for what I can do. Not to be belittled by what I can't do.

Here are the steps I have taken to recover;

1. I didn't accept "only the expert's opinions;" when in doubt, I found out on my own.
2. I didn't give up on myself and kept my grandson in my heart as my reason to get well.
3. I kept exploring ways to heal by stepping outside the box when needed.
4. I trusted myself, had the determination and curiosity to find out what was right for me.
5. I didn't take no for an answer, as I networked and kept asking for help.
6. What I truly knew grew from within. My old self was gone; I had to go through the grieving process, to allow my new self to emerge.
7. I had to trust the process and didn't let fear of the unknown get in the way of my recovery. I just kept thinking about what I was missing with my grandson and daughter.
8. I paid attention to my emotions. The right path felt clear and positive.
9. I went beyond book learning and logic and trusted my intuition. Intuition is real to me.

To know and not to do, is not yet to know! By an unknown monk

The gift from the accident is my uncanny ability to feel. When I touch someone or something my hands never forget. Feeling is my primary way of learning and remembering now. I've been known to feel earth quakes half way around the world. Tsunami's in the ocean, and the cries from the sea animals.

I have made lemonade out of lemons and have taught others to do the same. Setbacks are just warm-ups for success. My commitment and positive attitude are my gifts to myself.

Chapter 2

To Know and Not to Do

To know and not to do is not yet to know! By an unknown Monk

It's been my experience if someone is hurting, either physically or emotionally, it is impossible for them to make good decisions for themselves or their loved ones.

The following four courageous women were in a year study starting with 8 classes.

Each class was designed to their needs. Follow up sessions were conducted throughout the year. Continued instructions given where needed and was ongoing.

Let me introduce the four to you: Roberta, Vona, Anne and JC and "Courage" should be their middle name. Ladies, I have asked for your active participation all year long and I thank you. I challenged your long held beliefs and yet you stayed with me.

The English writer G.K. Chesterton said "The traveler sees what he sees; the tourist sees only what he has come to see" I asked you to view the teachings with the eyes of a traveler.

I offered you a new world of possibilities and you took up the challenge to explore them. You might have set out on this adventure with a different expectation other than what you experienced. I hope I have repaid your efforts many folds, offering you these skills to be the achiever you want to be. To those who shared their stories towards the end of the book: whether I have known you for 20 plus years or just a year or two; I Thank You, for continuing with your tune-ups!

The Optimist Creed

Promise yourself:

To be strong that nothing can disturb your peace of mind.

To talk health, happiness, and prosperity to every person you meet.

To make all your friends feel that there is something worthwhile in them.

To look at the sunny side of everything and make your optimism come true.

To think only the best, to work only for the best and to expect only the best.

To be just as enthusiastic about success of others as you are about your own.

To forget mistakes of the past and press on to the greater achievements of the future.

To wear a cheerful expression at all times and give a smile to every living creature you meet.

To give so much time to improving yourself that you have no time to criticize others.

To be too large for worry, too noble for anger, too strong for fear, and too happy to permit the presence of trouble.

To think well of yourself and proclaim this fact to the world, not in loud words, but in great deeds.

To live in the faith that the whole world is on your side, so long as you are true to the best that is in you.

Christian D. Larson: Published in 1912

Chapter 3
Roberta's Story

Her affirmation
*I free myself from faulty thinking and embrace productive thoughts.
I affirm the fresh choices that are possible and my responsibility toward
others is in supporting them in their choices.*

An animated 58 year-old single woman entered the classroom
determined to learn as much as she could that day. She cried
out "teach me all you know about how my brain works" her brain
health was the most important reason for being in class. Very
intelligent and well educated is just partly describes who she is,
but humor takes her farther more in life than her intelligence.
She's a true comedian. Roberta even looks the part, in dress and
facial features. She is just cute! When you look at her, you can see
that the top of her head is tilted to the left, and her chin is tilted to
the right. When I first met Roberta I told her that if I did nothing
more, my goal was to get her head on straight. We both laugh,
but I was serious and she thought her head was on straight! Just
recently she showed me a family group picture and tears filled her
eyes as she said," I now understand what you were saying seven
years ago about my head not being on straight. I finally can see
it." I have seen this often, people think they are standing straight
or laying down straight when they are not. Our brain and body
work funny that way. By the way, in the seven plus years that I
have known Roberta, her head is now straighter than it has ever
been. Roberta broke her left collarbone in an auto accident when

she was eight years old. Her head became pinned between the front two bucket seats of a VW bug. Even though she was treated for a broken collarbone; wouldn't it make sense that her head and neck would have been compromised? However, she was not treated for anything other than her broken collarbone. Until these classes, none of the attendees had equated an accident with a brain injury. Of course today, 50 years later, she probably would at least have been examined for a brain injury. Keep up the good work Roberta!

Roberta stays very active as a massage therapist and care giver. She meditates two hours a day; once in the morning and again in the evening.

As I see her, Roberta is unable to relax. She is easily startled, being a worrier. At times she feels insecure and nervous, a factor when she is in large crowds of people. Here come her animation and gestures, she taps her toes and her hand trembles as she becomes a nervous little fairy toe dancer.

Roberta describes having a life changing experience about 24 years ago, a nervous breakdown. Roberta's relationship of 14 years came abruptly to an end. She and her partner had a commercial cleaning business in which she worked side by side with him. Then she came home to care for him and his daughter doing most of the cleaning and cooking, as most women did back in the day. Never gotten married, when he wanted out of the relationship the only thing she asked for and walked away with was a bamboo coffee table.

Roberta thought she was dealing with the breakup fairly well. About four months later, but finding herself all alone she landed in the hospital suffering with hallucinations and a mental breakdown! Who wouldn't have some kind of life setback? You probably know someone who has had an experience like hers. Left with no money, no home, no family, wondering what life was all about. She was first diagnosed as depression induced psychosis. At some point her diagnosis was changed to being bi-polar. The mental health field is better than it was at the turn of the century, but there is still a lot of guess work involved, and medication is often the first and only mode of treatment.

Roberta was given no counseling back then, just drugs. Twenty four years has passed, but she continues taking the following medications. Clonazpan, Lamectal and Invega. Some of the side effects of Clonazpan are confusion, dizziness, drowsiness, depression, and hallucination, loss of memory, behavioral problems, and difficulty in breathing, swallowing, thinking and remembering. Lamectal side effects are; severely uncoordinated, rash, chest pain, digestive problems, dizziness, double vision, drowsiness, clumsiness and unsteadiness, poor coordination, anxiety, depression. Invega medication side effects are reaction to the injection site, sleepiness, feeling inner restlessness, tremors and shaking, shuffling, uncontrolled and involuntary movements, and abnormal movement of the eyes. It is apparent in her every day living she shows signs of involuntary muscle movement, joint pain and anxiety. Luckily, Roberta does not have all of the side effects from these three medications, but she does have more than she wants.

Lucky for her and with the assistance of her doctor and psychologist, the above medications have been reduced by 3/4 of what she was taking when the classes started. The tremors have been reduced, due to less medication. She calls me her healing coach and a friend who has provided her with tools, constructive information and affirmations. Her favorite positive thought, "I'm in charge and I am healthy."

Now, she experiences some normal thoughts and feelings that she did not experience in the past 24 years. Roberta is learning various tools to help her become healthier and learning to normalize her emotions successfully, as each day is a new found adventure and she is looking forward to her healthy future.

As an adult, Roberta has been to an emergency room twice because of head injuries; plus, her VW bug accident when she was eight years old. She's endured two whip lashes and, now has the physical signs of tremors, which her doctors described and diagnosed as a side effect of her medications. She has a low tolerance to light and noise, she also suffers anxiety and difficulty concentrating.

One may wonder how she could live a normal life. How does she work to support herself with all her health issues? I am sure it can be very difficult for her at times. You wouldn't know what she goes through each day, just by looking at or talking to her. She never complains, unless I pry it out of her. She doesn't blame others for her misfortunes. Sometimes we talk about what is considered "normal" from our point of view and what it means to her. I will give her, a suggestion or tell her stories just to get her thinking in a different way. My stories seem to work for her.

Roberta is the second child and the oldest girl out of five children. One brother is two years older and a sister one year younger than Roberta. She had another sister four years younger. Roberta's baby sister passed away from SIDS at the age of six months. At that time Roberta was almost five years of age. Losing her baby sister was very hard on Roberta, as it was for the rest of the family.

After that loss, and when Roberta was five years old, the entire family went on a humanitarian assignment and moved to Ecuador for five years, they were on a program similar to Peace Corps. While in Ecuador her youngest brother was born. Roberta, being the oldest girl, took over the care of her younger brother and carried him around everywhere. She was referred to as "Big Mama" as she was only eight years old when he was born and small for her age. What's this "Big Mama" stuff? Her mother never seemed to get over the loss of her baby daughter and medicated herself with alcohol and prescription drugs. With grief she essentially quit being a mother. Roberta's father hired a maid to cook and clean.

Her father began to lose himself in his work, which continued after they moved back to the United States. Now in America there was no maid to cook and clean. The household chores fell upon the children. Roberta being the oldest girl was responsible for a lot of the work. She felt responsible for her mother's sorrow. She remembers being five years old and setting in church with her mother, who was sobbing uncontrollably. Roberta remembers an old woman of faith who was in church with them saying that it was only natural for a young child to be responsible for their parents suffering. This feeling of being responsible for her mother turned Roberta into believing she was responsible for others as well, which has followed her throughout her life. For the longest time, she believed she was responsible for causing others unhappiness. Thinking it was her fault if things did not go well for them. She has always been empathetic, sensitive and able to feel other people's feelings. This grew into a sense of responsibility that was out of proportion, always thinking herself at fault and beating herself up for other's misfortune or pain and suffering. She has learned over the years that it is their life, not hers, and she is not responsible for others. She has a big heart and lives with compassion for herself and for others. She has dedicated her life to the healing of others. In more recent years, Roberta has focused on her own healing and doing the difficult work of coming to a sense of self acceptance. This is something her mother was never able to do for herself. In some ways she feels she is here to heal the female family lineage by healing herself.

When Roberta was in college she thought of sacrificing her degree, so she could be close to her mother. Becoming her mother's caregiver, knowing her mother was always better when Roberta was around. But, her mother encouraged her to stay in college by saying, "You have to save yourself child." This helped give Roberta the motivation to stay in school. She took pre med classes along with environmental and marine biology sciences and graduated with a Bachelors Degree in science. She also, spent 18 months going to college near Mexico City.

Roberta's story about her grief

Six months into this new found healing of hers, she experienced the death of a man for whom she was a care giver for a few hours a week. She had to assist him with his shopping, cooking and cleaning. Roberta felt miserable and the grieving process was very hard on her. She is very intuitive and trusts her intuition. When she last saw him she felt something was going to happen to him. Days later he died of natural causes. She's had these feelings before but, this time it scared her. We talked about her feelings as she was grieving over his passing and the conversation lead her into several other losses for which she began grieving all over again. Grief comes and goes in waves and those waves come when we least expect them.

There are three practices Roberta does to help with her grief. #1 She will pray and meditate. #2 She will take time for herself; quiet down and may remain quiet for several days, not hiding, just reflecting. #3 Write her "Dear Roberta or someone else's name" letter.

At the time of her client's death, Roberta's Father had a mini stroke. She told me her father was her rock and she really needed him. However, it has been difficult to visit him during her grieving process. Roberta has been praying for her father's recovery, as well. Losses are hard for everyone, even a near loss. However, she wrote her Dear Roberta's, Dear Father's, Dear Client's and even Dear Baby Sister and Dear Mom. All of her "Dear" writings have helped her through this grief process.

More importantly for Roberta, she has found that casting out any thought of disease or illness, plus not to "own it!" has helped tremendously. Her goal is to eliminate all antipsychotic medications with the assistance of her health care professionals.

About 17 years ago, Roberta followed the path of her guru who teaches the importance of meditation, prayer and being of service. This, she believes, along with a faith in God, aides her and is key for making it possible to have lasting healing results.

Nine months into her healing, Roberta writes; "What Linda has shared has been irreplaceable to me. I feel the tools, such as the daily gratitude's, the good deeds and Dear Roberta's have benefited me the most." I admit that sometimes I haven't been able to do these in writing, but when I can't, I just think what I am grateful for or what good deeds I have done; by doing so, I feel lifted up. They keep me thinking towards remaining positive. The "joy bank" and focusing on joy and fun have been great in terms of experiencing happiness and turning my mind toward a more positive outlook. Addressing more positive thoughts has given me a chance to reduce my thoughts of beating up on myself. My habits of negative thinking and beating up on myself have been very difficult to break, but I am on my way to releasing negativity."

Roberta's healing story in her own words

A couple of days ago, as I was helping a friend lift a storage container over my head, I experience an injury to my deltoids and rotator cuff. I knew it probably was a tear in the muscle.

As a massage therapist for more than 20 years, I have had many experiences helping others with similar tears. I had been under a lot of stress; I was experiencing car trouble with my clutch and /or transmission. Every time I went to get an opinion on the origin to the problem and how to fix my car, the symptom eluded the mechanics.

That night, my neighbor offered to work on my shoulder, which helped tremendously. My sister reminded me to put ice on the injured area and take ibuprofen for the swelling; advice I had given many times but somehow, when I was injured the healing tool went out the window.

A girlfriend stopped by to say Hi, and ask how I was doing. I explained what had happened and I must have unconsciously divulged my fears about not healing from this tear. She said it sounded like I was planning on being sick and could I be thinking about my funeral as well. It made me laugh at the foolishness of it, but she was right.

I have to say that the first thing I did when this injury came on, was to pray to God and I kept affirming that "God is/was healing me." This is what my spiritual teacher talks about and the disassociation from the pain and condition. I use this mantra or affirmation whenever I can remember.

The same day, there was another stress in my life. My 89 year old father was admitted to the hospital for double pneumonia and then the doctors discovered at that time, he needed a pacemaker. The next day, the author, Linda was going to be in the area, so I asked if she would work on me. I was full of pain and was thinking earlier in the day that I would never do massages again, or at the very least I'd have to have surgery. When Linda started to work on my body, she asked me right off the bat, what I was carrying on my shoulders. I said "I did not know but I would think about it." Also, she asked what I was thinking about at the time of the injury. I was not sure. As she worked on me, I started to cry telling the story about not being able to drive my car on the one hour drive to see my dad, and being reluctant to ask someone to drive me. When Linda said she would drive me, it caused a floodgate of tears. She told me, "One never knows when it is the last time one might see a loved one. You can't wait. Under these circumstances, you need to see your father today." All the while she worked on me she asked if I had used a water bottle behind my neck? I had forgotten about that tool, as well. I do know that the base of the skull is grand central station for the nerves coming out of the spine. Along with the cold water bottle and what she did to keep the swelling down, the lymph's had drained when she was done.... I was still in some pain and could not raise my arm yet. She told me that I had a lot of heat and energy in my shoulder area and I needed to take a look at what issues have been appearing to me that I needed to look at. Linda stated, "This situation usually appears in threes and has there been three kinds of these situations happening to you lately?" this question needed to be answered, but later.

Linda and I took the one hour drive to see my father, right then and there. Armed with a cold water bottle behind my neck and a cold pack on my arm, off we went. I now know that the cold behind my neck was responsible for the reduced swelling and my nerves getting the message that I could heal. I only spent about five minutes with my dad, since he just had surgery for the pacemaker earlier in the day, but it was such a relief to see him even for that short visit.

I wanted to get to the bottom of why this tear injury happened in the first place. I next used the "Dear Roberta" tool we learned in class. I verbally asked the questions as I was not able to write them down because of my injured shoulder. So I asked "Dear Roberta why did you injure yourself?" and "Dear Roberta's right shoulder why did you get injured, and why do you hurt?" I repeated any combination of these questions over and over.

What came up for me was the fear that my two dear friends and my father might be getting ready to make their transition. I could not bear the thought of losing them like I lost my mother earlier in life. The thought came that I had to bear the responsibility for each of them; not allowing them to chose for themselves. This thought has followed me ever since I was eight years old.

Being injured made me more open to receiving help from others, but I am also more determined to not be handicapped. I made the decision to do everything I could to help myself... I believe that God is absolutely responsibility for my healing, but I must do my part! "God helps those who help themselves" is something I have always thought was true.

As I was visiting my neighbor at the end of the third day and

I checked in with my arm, which was easily 200% better, she reminded me that dis-ease is about fear, (false evidence appearing real). I was aware of the energy that Linda had spoken of earlier and that I was holding it in my shoulder. Knowing that it was just fear allowed me to let it go. An incredible feeling of warmth and wellbeing came over my shoulder area. That night I saw a tattoo on TV which reminded me, it read "don't always believe what you see." This was a reminder to not buy into the appearance of illness and remember the truth about my wholeness.

This whole experience has given me a renewed desire to want to be committed to my own healing and wellness. A big part by using what Linda has taught us was about eating healthier. For me, it is more protein, more veggies and more complex carbohydrates, along with fruit, and more exercise. I have a renewed commitment of getting up from my chair and moving every half hour, like I used to. I am looking forward to practicing all of the many tools she has taught me with greater faithfulness and zeal. I have had a personal experience seeing how dramatic the tools work.

Conclusion

Since the classes started I have seen Roberta able to maintain a healthier lifestyle and move towards becoming more disciplined in practicing the tools laid out for her.

There are times when Roberta has a thought she just cannot shake. It's like a dog with a bone. One method to learn is how to become "present in the moment" in order to detach herself from nagging thoughts. For example: when going for a walk notice the scenery describing her surroundings out loud to herself. Also, if she is talking to people, focus on what the other person is saying. If Roberta finds her troubled thoughts are running amuck she can acknowledge them by saying to herself, "Isn't that an interesting thought," and then letting it go like a balloon drifting off in the air or sending it off on a sailboat. Not to stuff her thoughts or make light of it but feel that thought.

Another way Roberta can utilize the tools, is to write her "Dear Roberta's." This has helped her to overcome problems of being timid and not being able to stand up for herself (allowing people to walk all over her). She is feeling more self confident and experiencing greater self worth. She is learning to speak her truth and put herself first. Along with this pattern of taking care of self, there is a bonus of being less angry and resentful. She notices other people are valuing her more because she values herself more.

Most helpful in building her self-esteem, is the ability to write a list of accomplishments that she is proud of. It could be something that she did during the day.... or a trait she sees in herself that she likes. It could be something like, "Dear Roberta, I'm so proud that you are becoming more positive and happier." Recently Harvard Business School did research and found that if you write down several of your greatest accomplishments before trying to solve a problem, you could be 160% more successful solving that problem. They found when trying to solve a problem the reasoning part of the brain reacts much like the legendary deer seeing the headlights of a car the deer freezes in place.

Diagnosed with bipolar disorder more than 24 years ago was the main reason she wanted to learn more about the brain and how it works. She wanted to have more control over her health, because it was becoming hard to live with the side effects of her medications.

Here are her following techniques to change her cellular memory;

- ⋙ Super Brain Yoga, do once daily to connect the brain and the body systematically.
- ⋙ Keep her brain balanced by whatever she does on one side, do on the other side.
- ⋙ Keep a calendar on how she feels, and her sleep patterns during the full and new moon.
- ⋙ Write her "Dear's" to release grief.
- ⋙ Daily write down; "I want" make a list of what she really wants. Write "Gratitude's" so she feels thankful of what she has. Write when she gives "anonymously" to give her a sense of joy.
- ⋙ Detox her scalp twice a week to improve hair health and may prevent her from further hair loss.

- Add 65 to 75 grams of vegetable protein daily since she has been a vegetarian for many years and needs to repair muscle loss plus improve brain function and may even prevent hair loss.
- Check pH level at least four times a week for many reasons and especially because she's a vegetarian.
- Do the colors and numbers daily it's an easy way to balance everything in her life.
- Review her 10 successful things she has done at least 4 times a week, or more as needed.
- Use the "5 Elements of Health" daily to balance her whole body by living with the seasons.
- Read over and learn more about her Western and Chinese Astrology. Learn how to value the twins of her Gemini sign, by understanding the importance of giving to herself first and then giving to others. Learn how to listen to her monkey mind as it can be an assistant to her. When in doubt review the movie "Inside Out."

Roberta has taken the classes to heart, or should I say, to health. She has been incorporating everything she has learned somewhere into her everyday life. When she feels she has mastered one of the techniques she moves on to another. She has taken what she has learned and has passed them on to others. All I can say to Roberta is, KEEP UP THE GOOD WORK AND CONGRATULATIONS!

Amy Poehler believes~

I like the person who commits and goes all in And takes big swings and then maybe fails; Who jumps and falls down! Rather than the person who points at the person who falls: and then laughs.

I totally believe this too.

Chapter 4
Vona's Story

Her affirmation

A folk story tells of a farmer who set out to dig a well. The ground was still dry about 15 feet down and he grew frustrated. He moved to another location and repeated the process two more times. Then his wife suggested he dig deeper right where he stood. He followed her advice and soon he found an abundance of water.

Vona, fit for the job, assisted me in all the classes. Each of us greatly appreciated her for doing so. "Restore and remodel" was her mantra throughout all the classes. As a 74 year-old, single woman living on her own, she was ready to make a difference in her health. She has mild point stabbing pain most of the time throughout her body. Some would call it fibromyalgia. She just calls it "traveling pain." An injured C7 vertebra has been caused by multiple whip lashes. Being a diabetic for many years, this disease is her top health priority. Her latest surgery was corneal transplants in both eyes which were successful, but took six years to complete. The lengthy time frame was a result of her diabetes. Vona fell down several times in 2014, due to sinus problems. With sensory and cognitive conditions, along with her sinus problems, the accumulated issues, overwhelm her.

Vona still works part-time for her church and is lucky the job allows her to work from home about 65 hours a week. Church is a warm welcome to her social life. She becomes a social butterfly - fluttering as she creates an inviting atmosphere, making everyone feel comfortable when she entertains. People, people everywhere a diversified group of friends are always around her, she's like a magnet when it comes to fun loving entertaining. With a heart of gold and because she entertains so much, she always keeps her living space neat and clean. In her fireplace, instead of a messy fire, it houses a perfect wee village equipped with teeny tiny lights. Her home is full of whimsical art, many of which are her own creations. Studies conducted on how important a social life can be on our health, could be written about Vona. Being the oldest living person left in her family and her children living out of state her church and neighbors are her family. Everyone in her life seems to value her. Being valued by others is the making of good health.

Vona tells her story

"I think mothers need to support their children; however, my mother's concern was not for me. After high school, mom had a problem with me going to regular college, even though I wanted to go. She always liked my hair and forced me to go to beauty school. (It was cheaper.) She always liked how I did her hair, so I guess something came out of it, mom's happiness.

I was a tubal baby! The doctors operated on my mother to remove me. However, during the operation they found I was both in and out of the womb, so they chose to save me instead. I had lots of problems growing up and didn't really get a handle on any of them until 8th grade; probably because that was when I started my period. Because of my dyslexia, Mother always called me dumb; dyslexia was not diagnosed back then, so I had to overcome this disorder on my own.

When mother was failing in health, I went to my parent's small farm to help out for three months before she passed. Because of this, I can now say I love her. Maybe not for the way she raised me but for who she was I love her. The experience lightened my spirit and I know my new found health has come from it. It started with the belief that I am NOT my ancestry. All of my immediate family had arthritis and now have all passed away. I am the only one left besides my two daughters. I feel I have been blessed – I didn't really get pain from the "A" word until I became 65 years old. I do not like to name my illness' and didn't for many years.

Vona's diabetic story

"I have been trying to reduce my insulin addiction for years. I have loved sugary foods all my life! My mother excelled in candies and baked goods. She also made 10 to 20 loaves of bread a week, which I would eat the center out of one, at least every month. I really don't have much power over sweets and the weight it puts on me! I have read research that shows excess body fat is the most significant cause of type 2 diabetes.

I have lost major weight twice before. Once when I was around 30 years old, I got inspired and went on a week of strict vegetable juices to reduce the size of my stomach capacity. I slowly allowed myself to cook some vegetable combinations using lemon and pepper for spice. I ate just veggies and lost 30 pounds in 30 days. (I was younger and in good health then.) I lost a bit more before hitting 109 pounds. After seeing a picture of myself, I decided to gain six pounds to round it up to 115 pounds, which looked and felt better for my 5' 11/2" frame. I kept the weight off for 10 years. However, when I was 45, my thyroid went crazy and the emergency room staff couldn't find out why I had severe hypothermia my lips were blue, and my temperature was extremely low. After gaining 40 pounds, which I still haven't lost, the doctors diagnosed me with a thyroid disease.

In 2007, I began preparing for corneal transplant surgery in both my eyes. My blood glucose was so high, it took six plus years to heal my eyes. Because I was serious about reducing my glucose to heal better, I went on a raw foods diet. My surgeon kept asking me why I wasn't healing faster. Raw was great, I lost 35 pounds, and I reduced my glucose. While starting the vegetarian raw foods diet, I had proper support from my diabetic doctor. He even came to my home and gave a class for me and my friends on how to get enough protein on a vegetarian diet.

It's been seven years since I've been off raw foods and my weight has come back to a startling 195 pounds. In my head I haven't allowed myself to go past 200 pounds. At the start of these classes my A1c blood glucose level was at 8.2. I went to a nutritionist recently, where she recommended reading Dr. Fuhrman's new book: The End of Diabetes. I am not rushing into the diet because I don't have the support that I had before. However, it has only been a month, and I have reduced my Lantus, long acting insulin, by six units, and the insulin I take before meals, Humalog, has been reduced considerably and some days I take very little. Eating plant based nutritional foods is Dr. Fuhrman main premise. Since the classes, follow ups sessions and after considerable persistence by being mindful of my health, my A1c has dropped from 8.2 to 6.9 and I have started to see my waistline again. I am smiling!

When I need strength for a new adventure, like getting off insulin, I look towards my great, great, grandmother Elizabeth and her survival story and courage. She came alone to America, in 1860, with three small children, starting from Cape of Good Hope, South Africa. On the ship, to purchase her and her kids passage, she worked as a nanny; then in New York she worked again as a nanny to pay for her passage to St. Louis. It was there she joined a Mormon Wagon Train going to Utah and started walking across the plains. With her children by her side and all of her worldly possessions filling her handcart, Elizabeth left with 168 people; like her, most were pushing handcarts

The journey was treacherous walking and pushing handcarts across the plains, many people died on the way. My great, great grandmother's St. Louis to Utah journey, lasted seven month and went without sleeping in the same place twice. They were trying to beat the coming winter weather so they pushed hard. I don't know how she did it, but she pushed a handcart with three kids, nine, five, and four years old, across the plains, rivers and eventually across the Rocky Mountains. She went through two pairs of sturdy shoes and on the last leg of their journey she and her kids were barefoot. Handcarts are not like wheel barrels. You stand behind a wooden bar and push or pull your cart over uneven ground, not roads, full of your worldly goods in all kind of weather.

Arriving in Utah, she again worked to feed her children. A man had lost his wife and needed help with his seven children once again she became a nanny. Eventually, they married and had six more children. Between the two of them they had seventeen children, ten of which she birthed.

So if my great great grandma Elizabeth can be that strong, so can I. In fact, the year Obama became president his slogan was "I Can." So I attached a small sign to my office door that reads, "I CAN." I believe we all can, if we just get out of our heads and don't say: I don't feel good today or I will do it tomorrow, but tomorrow never comes. I'm not making light of my addiction to sweets for I know I have a long road ahead, but, as I said earlier, I am excited with my prospects!

Conclusion

Vona does not like to write in a journal as a daily practice, but has seen the positive results that the others have had. They all do the; I wants, gratitudes, the 10 successes often. The others write their Joys and put them in their Joy Bank. Surprisingly enough, Vona has made a beautiful Joy Bank but it's still empty. She does the colors and numbers faithfully and sees positive results. She helps others by teaching them to use colors and numbers as well. Her water intake, having to go the bathroom often and sometimes in a hurry, has changed. She has found that sipping water all through the day keeps her more hydrated and drinks most of her water before 3 pm. She goes to the bathroom less frequent both during the day and at night. Her cold water bottle is at her bedside every night and when needed she puts it behind her neck. She has found she has less sinus problems by using it. Her sinuses have been a problem since childhood but not so much now. Super Brain yoga has given her more mobility and flexibility with less pain in her joints and muscles. She once worked for a chiropractor and understands about the nerves and how they correspond to the spine. So the spine chart has been a good reminder.

Vona states "I am excited about the results of everything I am doing and I look forward to my future."

Vona, keep up the good work. I know it has been hard work getting your A1c down, but you have done it and soon it will be even lower. You didn't get to be a diabetic in a day, so you can't expect to get over it in a day. You are a very intelligent woman who has the guts and stamina to keep up your courage. Just like your great, great grandmother did when she took her family (your family) to a better life in a new country. If she could do it you can do it! I am sure as you change your diet, and work some of the other lessons, you have learned, you will feel better and have a life full of adventure. I believe that the TBI screening form should be given your doctors. How can anyone decide what health issue needs to be addressed without knowing the possibility of a TBI. Please think about giving it to your health care professionals, as you well know all of our body parts are connected and our brain is our master computer.

It's amazing how your skin glows and that sparkle is back in your eyes. Pat yourself on your back, keep up the good work, smile and praise yourself. You deserve a BIG CONGRATULATIONS!!!

Here are her following techniques to change her cellalar memory.

- ⇛ Super Brain Yoga, do once daily to connect the brain and the body systematically.
- ⇛ Keep your brain balanced by whatever you on one side, do on the other side.
- ⇛ Write her "Dear's" to release grief.
- ⇛ Get up every half hour and move your body.
- ⇛ Use a golf ball at least once a day to reduce tingling.
- ⇛ Use the cold water bottle behind neck for sinus problems.
- ⇛ Use colors and numbers to help ease stress in your body..
- ⇛ Incorporate your successes as a template regularly.
- ⇛ Check your pH level at least four times a week.

Chapter 5

Anne's Story

Her affirmation
My enjoyment of giving and receiving love, which leads me to participate in living life to its' fullest. I revel in the power of Divine love!

Anne walked into the first class late; never meeting me before, but she knew and trusted the others. She was never going to be late again! It was time to change by making connection in her life, and she knew it. A single woman in her middle 50's still, working full-time as an accountant she came with a career mind and enthusiasm. She questioned everything going on in that first class, but still completed all of the health questionnaires, even though she did not know why they were important. In fact, it took her several classes before she understood why those forms needed to be completed. I was not just teaching classes to create a healthy body; I was there to give tools to create a better balanced life, which included a healthy body and much more.

Her left knee was injured in a boating accident when she was younger. Placed in ICU with a life threatening flesh eating bacteria, Anne has changed her view point on death and living. Diagnosed with chronic pain syndrome, in addition to having fibromyalgia, has not been easy for any kind of recovery. She has medium pain intensity most of the time, including moderate headaches. However, she still is able to fully concentrate. Anne is a big teddy bear at heart, but her presence is professional. In each class, she reminds us that she has lost everything and at times questions, what is her purpose in this life. I often see, men and women in their middle 50's, questioning who they are and what is their purpose in life! When we are young, we find love, get married, have children, work hard, plan for retirement. Then, there is a loss of a job and income our only alternative is to sell the house. Our kids think we have become a failure. They may not want us claiming an excuse when their life is rotten as a result. Blame, blame goes with pain. Pain pain, go away!

Anne, in her middle 50's, has many more years to live. She expresses that she wants to move ahead, but her actions show her depression has frozen her. The main claim she had for bad health was her depression. I asked her, "Do you need your depression?" She explains with full intensity "My grandmother was depressed. My father was depressed. I am depressed, and my 2 kids are depressed. Depression runs in my family and I can't do anything about it." Again I ask "Can you live without your depression or do you need it?" After asking that question in several different ways, I finally gave up. For now, depression is a part of her life and she couldn't begin to think about life without being depressed.

Slowly, in each class, I introduced how the brain works to create depression, and added many tools to help with some forms of depression. She did not move fast, but every once in awhile, she would wade in and get her feet wet by using a tool here and there. Living around four generations of depressed people, questions must come up around what a healthy life looks like without depression. Question: Could I really do something about my depression? How hard would it be? Do I really want to do the work? What if none of the tools work for me? Depression is a big elephant to eat; it is hard, but many times it is worth it.

One needs to stay on course. It can be just as hard as going on a diet to lose 100 pounds, and keeping it off. It is hard but it can be done. There are professionals, who can help, as can; medication, counseling and techniques in this book, but none of them are easy. Freud likened depression to grief. The two are the same. The opposite of depression is not being happy, but being vital and worthy. Depressed people feel devalued. Anne, I want you to know you are a valuable person to me.

Back pain is associated with depression and one may get a better night sleep if their back doesn't hurt so much.

Sometimes, Anne suffers with sciatic pain and cramping in her right leg and buttocks; including muscle leg cramps at night. She also has lived with constant ringing in her ears. Anne also has dry skin, burning feet, itching skin, and the skin peels on the souls of both her feet she says it is due to hypothyroidism. She gets hives and her hair falls out, which is getting noticeably thin. She excessively worries and has a feeling of insecurity.

To get relief from her restless leg syndrome and burning feet, Anne used the cold, hot, cold, hot, cold soak, by putting her feet in salt water above her ankles, in the bathtub. She found it was was much easier than using the bathtub than using the bowls I recommended. The salt water soaks not only help her restless leg syndrome, it also helps her sleep better at night. This cold hot cold hot cold salt soak routine is very relaxing to the entire body.

Four months into the research, she told her best friend she felt uneasy about her job. It was hardly paying her bills and little money for anything else. She was just getting by. She was working with people she would not even enjoy socializing with and they had nothing in common. She thanked her friend for listening to her, sharing her feelings. Anne had a real problem doing the exercise "What do I want?" She believes that a person should never phrase their request as "I want", because the Universe gives us what we ask for and she didn't want to stay in a place of perpetual wanting rather than knowing and accepting her good. She phrased her requests, instead, with "I see." The very next day, after telling her friend about how she felt about her job, she was fired.

Getting fired for the first time can be devastating to a person. She had all the normal feelings of being fired, plus the questions: What was she going to do? She didn't have next month's rent. Would she become homeless or live out of her car? Surprisingly, within a week she could see some benefits of losing her job a month before Christmas. Why do so many people lose their jobs just before Christmas? Why do companies think they are doing people a favor by letting them go at the happiest time of the year? One week later, she had an interview for a new job.

We talked about some of the things she learned in class that would get her through it all. Remember, depression was one of the things she and her family have had to deal with all her life.

We talked about the tools: Dear Anne's, her joy bank, and her gratitude's along with some stretching exercises she could do before getting out of bed in the morning. I wondered, was her depression going to get her down this time, or would she be able to use some of what she learned to keep her spirits up? What was her color and number for the day of her interview? Anne responded, "Orange" but I don't have anything to wear that is orange." Her friend Vona gave her an orange pin she could wear, but if she wore it, she could not see it. So she decided to pin it on her purse and put the purse in front of her where she could see it throughout the entire interview. She had one more interview, with the other partner a day later, and this time she was wearing yellow, Voila! She had a job in time for Christmas and next month's rent. She loves her new job and they are impressed with her accounting and people skills. The company is owned by two intelligent men and there is a promising future for her.

Anne's personal story in her own words

I was born in Wyoming and had an idyllic childhood, although I suffered from chronic ear and throat infections. I was treated with an antibiotic called Achromycin, which has been linked to birth defects and tooth staining. The family moved to the Pacific Northwest when I was seven. Other than premenstrual depression, I had no major illnesses during my teen years.

I was in a car crash when I was 21 years old. I lost control on black ice and hit a loaded school bus head-on. I went through the windshield and suffered broken ribs, lacerations and bruising, but was never treated for a head injury.

I married and became pregnant in 1983. A few weeks into the pregnancy, my left eye lid began to droop. The pregnancy was miserable and I was very sick. The drooping eye lid went away, without treatment, by the second trimester. About two months after the birth of my daughter, I became very weak and depressed. The general muscular weakness increased until I was unable to care for my daughter. I was certain that I had thyroid disease, because both my father and grandmother had the disease. The doctors kept assuring me that I was testing within normal ranges. Both the muscular weakness and depression increased, until I was barely able to function. I was misdiagnosed with all of the following: a tumor on the thymus gland, a brain tumor, multiple sclerosis, lupus and finally myasthenia gravis (a fatal disease in which all muscle control is lost). This misdiagnoses made me so depressed. My internist finally conceded, I could try antidepressant medication and he prescribed 200 mg. of Elavil daily. I later found out that that amount was enough to knock out an elephant. I couldn't wake up and felt like I was in a constant fog. By this time, my daughter was 11/2 and had completely bonded to my mother as her primary care giver.

My husband took me to the beach for a much needed get away weekend. While sitting on a log looking at the ocean, I told God that I was no good to anyone and just wanted to die. I heard a small voice in my head tell me clearly and firmly, "Live your life as if you're well and you will be." Wow, what a concept! Take back control of my life! When we got home from the beach, I went to a book store to look up my symptoms in a PDR. The pages of the book turned to "Hyperthyroidism...and the words "may cause muscular weakness of the arms and legs" and "depression" hit me like a ton of bricks! I called the doctor and he finally prescribed a thyroid blocking hormone. After one month on the medication, I was vacuuming my floors, caring for my child and ready to go back to work. I started on a different antidepressant medication and felt wonderful.

I felt good until 1991, when my 2nd child was born. Following his birth, I suffered from extremely debilitating arthritis (migrating to different joints) and giant, platter sized hives. I was diagnosed with chronic pain syndrome, commonly known as Fibromyalgia. After seeing countless doctors and trying every antihistamine available, I had no diagnosis for the chronic hives (idiopathic) and NO symptom relief. I suffered with the hives daily for 18 years. I finally saw an allergist who specialized in hives. The treatment was easy! For the past six years, I have taken two 10 mg. Claritin daily for complete hive control. No hives!

In 1996, I had surgery to remove my gallbladder and in 2007, surgery for kidney stones. In 2007, I was in a boating accident and suffered a torn meniscus, which couldn't be repaired surgically.

I had to use a wheel chair for four months, and after hours and hours of physical therapy began to slowly walk again.

I escaped a domestic violence situation with pretty much just the clothes on my back. I was unemployed, homeless and broke. I lost everything, including every friend and familial relationship that I knew. I found a place to live and got a job, but was so emotionally damaged that I cocooned myself from the outside world. I smiled at all of the appropriate times and sometimes even laughed, but inside I was suffocating in my inability to connect and relate to the world.

In 2012, I contracted a flesh eating bacteria. I had major surgery to remove the infected portion of the back of my thigh and spent 10 days in the ICU. It was a long road to recovery and it set me back in my health, emotions and finances.

Although I was intensely lonely, I couldn't trust myself to make good decisions about people and I couldn't trust people not to abuse me. I lived that way for almost four years until I just couldn't take the aloneness any longer. I found a church to attend and on the first day that I sat and listened to the speaker, I broke down sobbing, because it dawned on me that I wasn't just broken...I was shattered. Shattered beyond repair; so many fragments...no way to heal. I felt no hope, no life and no spark. The grief for my former life and the former 'me,' the strong version of myself that I liked, was so intense, it was palpable. I didn't know how to go on, or if I even wanted to. How do people cope with so much grief and despair? I didn't know if I had the strength to even try, but I knew I had to do something. I just didn't know what. I met a woman at church named Vona and she invited me to participate in a sense of mind, body and spiritual wellness classes that Linda was teaching and to participate in a year study. My main goal was not to heal my body, but to heal my soul. I needed to connect with people again. Really, deeply connect. And it has been a journey. Not always easy, not always fun, but always of benefit to me. A journey filled with discovery, self-awareness, laughter and tears. I've come a long way in the past year. We all have. We've developed a tight circle of friendship and formed deep and abiding bonds of friendship. I will always, always be grateful. Thank you Linda, for never giving up on us and always finding answers to any of our questions. Your faith and wisdom inspired me and is giving me hope for a brighter and healthier future.

Ten months after classes started, I developed shingles. Yuck! Painful! I suggest to everyone "Get a vaccination!!!!" see my story below:

I think I know the cause. I have been dealing with some deep and traumatizing emotional baggage in weekly therapy. It's not easy to have your life and all of your major big ticket mistakes up for scrutiny, judgment and analysis.

My case of Shingles started with excruciating pain on my left side, which centered around the rib cage. I have never felt that type of pain before. So I wasn't sure what was going on and just wished it away. By the next day, the pain was worse and it hurt to move or breathe. Vona (another woman in our class) happened to come over to my house and I showed her the strangely shaped rash that I had developed overnight. Just four little dots in a perfect square shape. Thank goodness Vona knew that I was developing "Shingles." I went to a local Urgent Care Center and was given a prescription for anti-viral medication and 5% Lidocaine gel. Off I went to the pharmacy, sure that I would be feeling much better in a couple of days. The anti-viral medication was only $20.00, but the numbing gel was $470.00!!!!! I had to settle for a much lower dosage (2%) and more affordable prescription of Lidocaine. Unfortunately, I didn't get a lot of relief from the Lidocaine. The following weekend I went to a drug store to look for an OTC pain cream. Their pharmacist was actually very helpful and when I informed her I couldn't afford $470.00 for 5% Lidocaine, she showed me to the hemorrhoid aisle. There on the shelf was 5% Lidocaine gel for only $33.00. Score!

By now the rash had fully developed and spread from my navel to my spine and from my bra line to my panty line which made wearing clothing unbearable! After about a month the rash finally started to clear up and is now only visible under the skin like a faint purple scar. But the nerve pain is chronic, severe and persistent. At this point in time, my alternatives were to trust conventional medicine and get a prescription for Lyrica (expensive and massive side effects), Anticonvulsant medication (mega-side effects) or tricyclic antidepressants (mega-mega side effects). None of those options sounded appealing to me. I decided to go the holistic path and started doing research. On the advice of one of Linda's professional friends, I started taking large doses of vitamins (15,000 mg's of Vitamin B-12 sublingually, 6,000 mg's of Vitamin C, 400 units of Vitamin E, 15,000 units of Vitamin D-3, and 2,000 mg's of L-Lysine) daily. I also found some Lysine cream, Vitamin A cream and Emu Oil at a Vitamin Store. I still have persistent nerve pain, but at least it is bearable and I am back wearing my normal work cloths. (No signs of the shingles to date, healed and Anne's life is back to normal).

I came to Linda's classes looking for spiritual wellness and a sense of connection. I found much more including four great friends. I practice many of the lessons. My favorites include: Colors and Numbers, Dear Anne's, the Gratitude's, Joy Bank, Chinese Astrology along with daily affirmations, cleansing with rubbing alcohol and the cold water bottle behind my neck and knees. We all now support each other and share our successes.

Conclusion

Anne may have taken baby steps at first but within a few months she was doing most of techniques I had assembled for her. She was good about asking questions and made us all think. Anne realizes that many of her difficulties steams from her auto accidents complicated by other health condition that her body has gone through. The accumulation of repeated health issues, numerous auto accidents including going through a windshield, could you have a TBI? Who knows, you have never been tested for a TBI. I suggest that you consult with your health care professional. Some researchers believe that fibromyalgia is caused from multiple traumas to the body resulting in traveling pain throughout the body, Anne you have had a combination of traumas which has made your health run amuck.

- ⇶ Massage at least once a month for improving your serotonin and melatonin levels.
- ⇶ Continue using Super Brain Yoga so your brain and body can understand how to function on it's own.
- ⇶ Use color in numbers to reduce your daily stress.

⇛ Review your 10 successful accomplishments on a regular basis.
⇛ Use cold hot cold hot cold sock on your feet each night to relieve restless leg syndrome and get better sleep, it's relaxing.
⇛ Read your affirmation daily.

Now having some great tools and slowly you can add more into her lifestyle. CONGRATULATION! Anne, pat yourself on the back seeing, your progress has made us all smile.

Have a Tea Party, a real tea party. Use a tea pot with a fancy little tea cup and saucer, not a mug. You may want to try Passionflower tea; this tea helps your brain make more calming hormones like serotonin. It works well for home bound people who have worries and thoughts rushing through their heads. Someday you may want to invite a friend to your tea party.

Play dress up. Go into your closet, look for something you have been saving all these years. It might be a scarf, a fancy belt, hat or a piece of jewelry. Use anything to get started, be a queen, a lady of the night, a fairy, try anything, you are just playing and no one can see you.

Think about the movies that use to make you laugh. Laughter is the best medicine. Now go rent some of your favorite movies and have a weekend of laughter. Do this laughter weekend once a month for a year. Twelve times of two days of laughter and you will be a different person in a year.

Don't remember how to play or never had time to play as a child. Don't worry; go and volunteer in a Sunday school class, help your friend when she babysits her grandchildren. These kids are not yours so it will be easy to learn how to play from them.

Think about the things that made you happy when you were young. Make a list of them and put them on your "Laughter Bucket List", keep adding to the list and do some of them often. Get some of your friends together and brainstorm, what makes each of you happy, they may remind you of the Good Old Days.

Chapter 6

JC's Story

Her affirmation

I am a person of high energy. There have been times I have pushed myself too near exhaustion. When this happens, I am guided to rest my weary brain and body. As I let go of the wall built from my "do-it-all-myself" attitude, the wall begins to crumble.

JC is not an open book. She thinks long and hard, processing her thoughts before speaking and carries herself in conversation, which is short in length, but deep, nonetheless. Smart looking, tall stately woman in her 70's, became retired after the crash in 2008. Moving from Silicon Valley in California to the Northwest has been a big adjustment on her. Living in separate houses, she and her husband live close to each other and are still on good terms with each other. When she leaves her home, you will find her smartly dressed in a professional manner. Everything about her appearance is in order. Underneath, and never expressing pain, she has an uncertain prognosis with her stage three kidney disease (due to hypertension). Plagued with seasonal depression, and sometimes neck and lower back pain these medical issues are another side of JC that she prefers not to show.

Strong light irritates her eyes and she gives two reasons for the problem. One, she has the beginning of cataracts in both eyes and two; she has light blue eyes which are more sensitive to light than darker eyes. This could be true! Or could the cause of her sensitivity come from another source? Her mother told her when she was a baby her dad dropped her on her head, or could it be because she was in three auto accidents? In one accident, she was rear ended and got a server whiplash and little medical attention. The other two, she was smashed on the right side and another smashed on the left side in a "T" bone style accident. During all of these accidents, her head was jostled, creating an accumulative effect that could cause a TBI. Any one, or all of these, could have caused a traumatic brain injury. After retirement depression became a problem. However, she finds comfort in opening the windows to allow fresh air to flow through the house. She has ringing in her ears and is sensitive to hot weather. She finds she gets keyed up easily and then she has a problem calming down has linked her to more depression. She can be highly emotional and this concerns her. Depression, anxiety, light sensitive eyes, ringing in her ears, mood swings creating a highly emotional state with difficulty calming down. Being in constant neck pain with perpetual discomfort has become her norm. Exhibiting low blood pressure and then high blood pressure off and on through her adult life and being medication for each. All of the above are indication of a having a brain injury.

Getting older and experiencing some female problems a partial hysterectomy was recommended. By having her gall bladder removed several years ago, her liver has to work harder to produce enough bile to digest her food. She is prone to diarrhea, as well as lower bowel gas several hours after eating. She gets a burning sensation in her stomach that eating can, sometimes relieve. Acid reflux upsets her throat, along with a nervous stomach. JC gets indigestion soon after meals. Once, she had a dislocated left shoulder, along with pain down her lower back to her pelvic area that continues to show up every once in a while.

While the cost of living is less in the Northwest, leaving what was familiar to them including long time friends, kids and grandchildren can be very problematic for many. Grandmothers need to be with their grandchildren and grandchildren can benefit being with their grandparents. The constant gloomy short days of winter can demolish any ideas of a happy and fruitful retirement for her.

The question is does JC have some of the effects of Seasonal

Affective Disorder? Not getting enough sunlight can affect our pituitary gland. Regular use of a light box can relieve this condition. Depression studies have found that creativity, sharing and giving helps with depression. Whether we are doing something by ourselves or collaborating with others in a creative way can help the body release dopamine which helps reduce the effects of depression. Creativity can be sparked through many forms. Among them: writing, drawing, painting, decorating, singing or gardening, cooking, and so on.

Recently she had her semiannual exam with her kidney specialist. She told JC she had several patients who had stage three kidney disease. Although some have had the disease for many years, they are doing just fine, as long as they keep up their exercise program and salt free diet. All have been living normal lives and she should expect the same. This was the first time JC heard that she could live a long, normal life. Her doctor hadn't given her this kind of encouragement before. Could you just imagine how relieved she must have felt hearing her prognosis? When she gave us the news we all wanted to celebrate with her. Smiles were on all of our faces. She was feeling the most positive about her health since the classes started.

She started doing her "Dear JC's" twice a week and by doing so she has gotten to know herself as a confident woman. Those "Dear's" have made her see herself in a whole new light and the light just radiates out into the world around her. It is so refreshing to see her in this new light. Now it is time to move on to the Dear kidneys or Dear pain in the neck. As she writes a page or two on each subject, she may find out why she has these health conditions. JC is always reading, studying and learning she has volumes of learning material on bookshelves, by her nightstand and in the office. Many of the volumes are on personal growth, alterative healing and spirituality.

When I emphasized the importance of writing down her gratitudes, she expressed how important they had already been to her; she has been doing them for many years. As she expresses herself, anyone can tell she is a very intelligent woman with a diverse background. She is full of information and others can learn much from her. She places golf balls in handy places throughout her home. When she needs one she can get to it easily. She has passed the importance of using the golf ball on to many of her friends, because of the pleasing effect it has on her. JC has been doing very well keeping a positive attitude and tries not to speak ill of others. Her personal philosophy is, what she gives out, will come back to her.

When JC came to class she came with her knowledge in tow; ready to learn what I had to teach and then blend the two together. Being a Cancer in Western Astrology and a Monkey in Chinese's Astrology, brought new insight but was sometimes hard for her to take in that information and use it. She wants to know more about the two types of astrology by blending the two together and can't wait until I have another class. You may have heard the old saying, "My monkey mind gets in my way and never stops." JC's monkey mind does act up but her cancer traits are grounding. JC is very much a family and community minded person she keeps very active in both. To know and not to do is not yet to know. She just needed to know a little bit here and there to get her going in the right direction towards choosing better health. Hopefully her monkey mind will not get in her way again while she is attempting to age with her purpose in mind.

Conclusion

JC does not need much, except for all of us to stay in contact with her from time to time. How do you eat an ELEPHANT? One bite at a time! When things get a little out of sorts for her, we will be there! At times, we all forget about what we know, especially when the pain gets out of control. Just a reminder JC, we are here for you if you forget and need to recall some techniques. We can't control the whole world, we can only control how the world tries to control us. Everyone needs a tune up once in awhile, and this year was JC's tune up time. Here are the following techniques to change cellular memory:

>>> Do something creative each week.
>>> Do your Dear's at least once a week.
>>> Continue using the golf ball for full body health.
>>> Continue using the water bottle behind her neck as needed.

- ⟫ Continue putting joy into your Joy Bank and go over them often.
- ⟫ Keep using the cranberry drink for your kidneys.
- ⟫ Add color to your wardrobe and display color on your upper body.

If she places messages of joy into her Joy Bank like a savings account, she can make a withdrawal whenever life gets her down. By reading the messages from time to time she will stay buoyant.

I suggest that Roberta and JC get together to share or fire off ideas by brain storming on how their monkey minds work in their favor and how they sometimes don't! Explore how each partakes in celebrating their monkey mind by taking full advantage of the chatter. JC keep up the good work in creating better health for yourself and your community. One final note, put some real play into each day. Move your body often and laugh a lot. You are a courageous woman, and I thank you for being a part of this year's assignment. What an adventure! CONGRATULATIONS! CELEBRATE! CELEBRATE! and CELEBRATE again! Do something exceptionally special for yourself!

Nerve Chart

Chapter 7

Built-in Physician

"Hidden away in the inner nature of real man is the law of his life... There is present in everybody a built-in Physician that can do the only perfect and complete job healing if we would but let it" by Ernest Holmes.

Researchers and health care professionals used to believe that a person's life was written entirely by the genes that they were born with. This was the health care philosophy until recently. New researchers have learned more about genetics, our biological inheritance, and more and more, they realized that for the most part our lifestyle decisions and our behaviors have far more impact on a healthy longevity than heredity. A person's genes defines their basic biology but our health decisions and habits control the way the genes will affect our body and health in general. If we lived by our genes alone, we would suffer from thousands of diseases experienced by our ancestors throughout out life, but we don't. Disease carrying genes are not our destiny.

A recent report states; "The environment in which you grow up in is as important as your DNA in determining the person you become. Certain genes can lead to vulnerability, but not inevitability." Our health decisions and habits can change by starting right now. I hear too often "I have always done it this way, so why should I change," or "My whole family has XYZ problems; it runs in my family." I'm not going to make anyone change if they don't want to. However, there are proven things available to us that we can do for ourselves. Sometimes it is hard to decide which one to do and what is good for us. There is so much information out there, it can be very confusing.

Our brain and body always moves as fast as today's technology moves. Did you know that?

Chronological age is not a biological age. We often will blame a health condition such as a bad shoulder, knee, or back, etc., on old age. If age was to blame, then it would stand to reason that both shoulders and both knees would be degenerated at the same time, not just one of them. These problems are due to cumulative stress and traumas, not the passage of time. Research has found that there is no natural aging process. Aging does not occur in all human populations at the same age. Science now knows that high blood pressure is not inevitable in the aging populations in some countries, as it is in America. In countries that are isolated from Western society, the elderly have the same blood pressure as their young. Western women have a problem with osteoporosis. However, women in other cultures around the world do not suffer from osteoporosis or similar degenerative disorders as western women. Why?

Time is not our enemy. Our choices in the way we live can be our enemy. The human body is an amazing collection of synergistic entities controlled by what can only be described as innate intelligence. The body is designed to be totally self-functioning and self-healing, if we only let it. We tend to think of healing when we suffer a cut finger or have a broken bone, but healing is a constant process of replacing old cells with new ones. For example, red blood cells are replaced at a rate of 100 billion a day as one trillion total red blood cells are in constant circulation. The body is constantly analyzing what is happening, both within the body and the environment outside the body. It makes adaptive changes as necessary.

Aging can best be defined as a gradual loss of the body's ability to respond to the environment. Aging is not just the effect of chronological time, but more so the abnormal stress we place on our body, which gradually breaks it down. Most of this break down is caused by inactivity, chemical pollution, (which include over the counter and prescription drug toxicity), plus neurological and postural stress placed on the body. Inactivity and disuse is deadly and many of our degenerative diseases that plague Americans are cause by an inactive lifestyle. It's time to get up and start moving. If you don't MOVE you will get run over!

Fifty percent of the decline in physiological function, which includes weak muscles, stiff joints, and low energy levels, is actually due to disuse and not to a normal consequence of aging. Without movement, the body and the brain will not be healthy. Spinal movement stimulates brain function in the same way that a windmill generates electricity for a power plant. Half of all the nerve pulses that are sent between your brain and body are in your spinal cord and are for the delivery of movement stimulation to the brain. This enables the brain to coordinate activities, such as concentration, learning and emotions with motor control and organ function. Movement charges your brain's battery and makes you able to think better, feel better and function better. All of this is essential to good health and longevity.

Movement is your choice. More people die from sedentary lifestyle than from smoking. The central nervous system regulates the aging process and is dependent upon healthy stress responses. Proper neurological signaling in the body is the primary key to psychological, emotional, hormonal, and immune system health and longevity. The quality of healing is directly proportional to the functional capability of the central nerve messages.

Until recently, there was a greater quantity of communication in the human body than in all of the manufactured communication systems in the world. That is before this era of high technological.

The coordination and precision of neurological and biological communication systems in the body is beyond most people's comprehension. Now, you can get a better idea of why I use today's technological communication industry as an example. You may not truly understand the human body, but it becomes easier to understand, as we have seen our lives changed by our current technology communication.

Our brain is the hard drive, and our mind is the software. As an example, if we were to use an accounting system and our hard drive could not handle the accounting system, what would we do? Our brain and body work together just as well as cell phones, laptops and computerized cars. What happens when our electronic devise have any of the following issues: virus, break down, overload or loss of a signal? We DO something about it. Our brain and body work or not work in a similar fashion. It is time to do something about your HARD DRIVE and SOFTWARE? We cannot trade our body or brain in for a newer or faster model. However, we can clean up the viruses (bacteria), hackers (improper foods and drugs), attackers (negative thinking and negative people), and low batteries (not enough sleep, rest, joy, social interaction, prayer or meditation). How often do you run your security system to make sure you are getting the best out of your electronic technology? How often do you check your body and brain systems?

I truly believe if you only have one way to do something, you're a robot. If you have only two ways to do something you're in a debt dilemma (a state of owing). I think you need at least three ways to do something before you have some sense of real flexibility and freedom. To really have a choice, you need at least three ways to do anything. In these writings I offered you a tremendous variety of new choices in various areas to improve your life. The choice is yours. I truly hope that from the stories of those courageous people and their journeys to better health, you will find a better health path for yourself. Don Juan once said "A path without a heart is never enjoyable, because you have to work hard to even take that path. On the other hand, a path with a heart is easy; it does not make you work at liking it." Before you even start taking a particular path, ask yourself "Does this path have my heart?" I hope that you have realized by now that I came with my heart, to join your heart as a kindred spirit and if you wish, our paths will cross again.

If you have found some way to take control of your life and health, and it works for you please continue using it. Also, if you are uncertain about any of the techniques in this book, please consult your health care professionals. From the stories in this book, I hope you will gain some information to help you take more control of your life and health.

Chapter 8
Where Attentions Goes, Energy Flows

A Native American Grandfather was teaching his grandchildren about the nature of Life on Mother Earth. He said to them. "A fierce fight is going on inside me. It is a terrible fight between two wolves. One of wolves is called Evil. He is fear, anger, envy, sorrow, regret, pride, competition, superiority and ego. The other wolf is called Good. He is joy, peace, love, hope, serenity, humility, kindness, benevolence, friendship, courage, empathy, nobility, generosity, truth, compassion, devotion and faith. This same fight is going on inside you, as well, as within every other person, too. The children thought about it for a while and then one child asked, "Grandfather, which wolf will win?" The Elder wisely replied. "THE ONE YOU FEED."

Wherever your attention goes, your energy flows. Likewise it is true that wherever your energy flows your attention goes. ATTENTION AND ENERGY TRAVEL TOGETHER. Energy gives LIFE to any thoughts you focus on. In knowing this, you can make wise choices and vow to maintain a positive point of view on all of your LIFE situations. So dream a BEAUTIFUL DREAM OF BEING THE BEST YOU CAN BE AT 100 YEARS OLD.

I recently gave a woman some easy steps to help herself, because she was complaining about losing her energy. She was about to turn 86 years old and reminiscing about all of the things and opportunities she had when she was young and no longer has today. She called me the next day and said "I just don't believe that anything you told me to do for myself will help me." My response to her was. "Then do not do them." She has the freedom to make choices for herself.

My advice to you, as you are reading this book, if you do not believe it will work, do not try it. Please consult your healthcare professional as soon as possible. The information in this book is not meant to replace any of your health care professionals or to replace any of the advice they have given you. It is to give you some information that can better assist you with the medical care you are now receiving. Plus it offers you ways to have a more balanced life.

You will find that the information you are about to receive from this book will help build cognitive reserves, so that the brain can keep the body balanced and healthier.

You will find from these powerful committed people, their stories and the path each one of them took. How they took inventory of themselves, their chartered course, making a better future for themselves. They decided where they want to go and the choices needed to fulfill their dreams. They are on an adventure to age with a purpose.

Their stories are not the standards of others who put the aging process into "Oh, you are just getting old" or "This is what happens to old people." They wanted to take control of their own aging process in their own way by having options.

Chapter 9

Self Compassion

Self compassion comes from our suffering; Self compassion equals real happiness. We wouldn't appreciate the light until we had been in the dark!

Almost everyone, probably without ever realizing it, thinks they have divided their lives into what they like and what they don't like, or what they want and don't want. They are doing both of these in many areas of their lives. However, most people probably haven't noticed that they can subdivide their likes and dislikes into what they would LIKE and what they would WANT.

We put on yellow color glasses in so many areas of our lives that it never occurs to us we can change the color of the glasses. Not realizing that those yellow color glasses just have not been working for us for a long time, we stay where we are or worse yet, stagnate and decay. For most, making changes comes only when something bad has happens that forces us to change. Why not make a choice to change BEFORE something bad forces us to change.

These courageous people have taken the challenge and changed their yellow colored glasses to purple, pink, blue or some other color until they found something that worked for them.

If you continue doing the same things that you have been doing all your life, you will only get more of the same. It is time to try something different. Oh, by the way, retirement or stopping work is not the change you need, especially if you have not found something to replace work when you retire. For many, after retirement their health declines or they even pass away soon afterwards. It may help to change to a job you actually love or find a rewarding place to volunteer. If you hurt, feel ill or have dementia, what can you do other than blame your pain or illness on why you can't have what you desire. STOP! Read these people's stories.

Get up, start moving, volunteer to help others, not because you have to, but because you want to. Notice the joy that you get by giving to a total stranger. Then give a total stranger the opportunity to feel that same joy, by giving to you. Smile and say Thank You.

Many of the teachings offered in this book and in my classes have no side effects. They have been tried, used and studied. Hopefully the information you need to make wise choices for yourself and your loved ones will be simply conveyed. I have only been the motivator by assisting these courageous people on their journey to a better way of ageing.

In their stories, they tell how they have regained their feeling of empowerment as they journey to a better life. This has given them a new way to live, to be happier and healthier until the age of 100 and beyond.

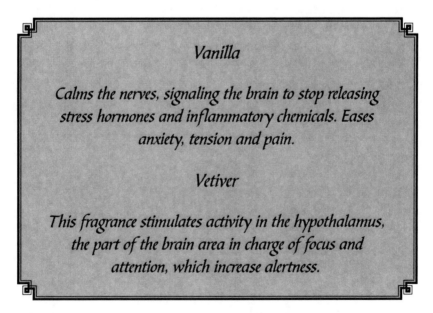

Vanilla

Calms the nerves, signaling the brain to stop releasing stress hormones and inflammatory chemicals. Eases anxiety, tension and pain.

Vetiver

This fragrance stimulates activity in the hypothalamus, the part of the brain area in charge of focus and attention, which increase alertness.

Chapter 10

My Body, My Brain

Just as a great distance is covered in many small steps, a great work is the culmination of many small acts of kindness, compassion and generosity. Give these as well to yourself!

As a human being, we have a physical nature, a mental nature and an emotional nature. Our physical nature is expressed in many ways, such as, sharing an authentic smile to someone or a sincere hug with family and loved ones. Our mental nature is expressed by thinking loving thoughts of wholeness and abundance, and by showing compassion and understanding to ourselves and others. Our emotional nature expresses love by forgiving ourselves and forgiving others, by releasing attachments to the past and holding hope for the future.

Some days we may forget to take care of our body or our brain, but our brain and body never forget to take care of us. It spontaneously pumps blood, digest food, inhales oxygen and exhales emit vapors. Our brain allows us to be able to speak and make decisions. Our brain communicates with every cell of our body, all day and night without us even thinking to do so.

I am amazed by the workings of my brain and my body. It renews itself and responds to my choices. Whether I realize it or not, my life is in motion within me. I stretch my muscles and as I do, I feel energized and renewed. Each and every day I make a conscious choice which will affect my health and the vitality of my body. This is my commitment to myself,; the better I am to myself, the better I am to those around me. Often times, I remind people that, first you have to take care of yourself, so you can take care of others. An airplane is an example: when ready for take off, the flight attendant will give you these instructions, "If your oxygen mask drops down, first put it on yourself before helping others." I remind people over and over, we need to take care of the caregiver first, so the caregiver can give.

Words have a powerful life of their own, each emitting their own energetic vibration. When combined with intent of the user, work can bring a new level of meaning to the reader, even if it is on a subconscious level. Words carry, within their letters, the secrets of their fuller meaning, to those who are open to receiving the information. Words reveal many truths that are contained within them. I encourage you to read this book with open eyes and heart, to receive all the blessings contained within this book, and through these powerful courageous people's experiences.

We are all in the same boat, regardless of our path. We all have a mind, we all possess an ego, and we all hear voices urging us towards either the high road or the low road in our life decisions. Regardless of the spiritual traditions we each follow, the terrain is the same. Although the names given to trials and tribulation may differ, they will still challenge us. The rewards may be referred to by different names, but they will inspire us just the same. I ask that you birth within yourself the purest qualities of compassion, love, respect, strength and faith in yourself first and foremost. All this leads us to exist in a balanced way of life.

Every spring I have faith that the air will begin to warm and new sprouts and blossoms will appear. This has happened every spring before now and it will happen every spring to come. With this same faith, when I am hungry, food will be available. When I am thirsty, my thirst will be quenched. When I am cold, I will have shelter and clothing. As I become aware of these statements, I am able to drop my worries about what is to come. I let go of any fear and anxiety about my future and rest on my unwavering faith. I am then free to move toward the things that I fear and take action I need to take. I do not have just one action to choose from, but many clear cut actions that are positive for me. I am constantly learning to combat automatic negativity that comes my way and could make me feel bad which interferes with the health of my brain.

Changing Brain

Technology makes it possible to engage in multiple actives at once. I may eat while talking on the phone, or check my emails while eating. Multitasking keeps me from being fully present in each activity and leaves me feeling disconnected. Mindfully awake, I embrace my connection with life. One task at a time!

In recent years there has been much research on the brain that has proven we can create a better brain no matter where our brain is now. The brain can be changed. Research has proven that we can create a healthier brain, if we work at it. Each day, I personally work on balancing my brain, body, diet and emotions. Each day, I am getting better and better. This brain of ours keeps our body, emotions and thinking balanced and working properly, if we allow it to do so. Why wouldn't we want to keep our brain safe and healthy at all times!

Our brain is constantly sending messages to other parts of our body, three times faster than a fast ball in the game of baseball. So how is your brain doing right now? We can actually train our mind to reduce stress in our life, and by doing so, it takes our brain in a different direction. Where the brain, goes the body tends to follow. Some people tend to wake up each morning, already mentally exhausted from thinking of what they need to do today, or what they forgot to do yesterday. All of this cluttered thinking is going on in their conscious mind, and while they are physically getting ready for the day. It's too much for their brain and body to handle.

The nerve circuits in our brain, trip alarms. The alarms set off, in a not so rested body, to charge ahead and GO right now! The alarms set off hormones to get the heart pumping faster, the immune system to slow down its patrols for invading pathogens. Our muscles pull in more oxygen, ready for action, and our senses go into high alert. All of this happens on a relatively normal day in our Western Society.

Now, just imagine the toll that stress can take over time on our body. Unchecked, stress and the metabolic changes can cause serious ailments; such as, obesity, heart disease and high blood pressure, to name a few. Long-term stress also runs down the cell tissue in organs that causes them to age before their time. We clearly need to add brain fitness into our life style, the same as we do diet and exercise. Researchers say that the mind can triumph over matter, harness it well and beat sickness and pain. In Western Society, on average, our brain at any given time is balancing 150 uncompleted tasks and 15 unaccomplished goals. This causes much stress on our body. These days, we have new technology that will allow us to take a look at what stress and worry actually looks like in the brain.

In one study a functional magnetic imaging (MRI) was used. The MRI captured real time changes in oxygen flow in the brain during mental tasks, to map a baseline state of cranial activity. They found the amount of oxygen expanded during many routine chores. The MRI painted the brain working, by trying to tie up a bunch of loose ends, when the brain was under stress. The brain, in the process of going through the days "to do list", had activated a particular current of neurons that looped the hypo thymus, pituitary and adrenal glands, and triggers the release of the hormone, cortisol. This example is much like the action of a pebble dropped in a pond. The circuits turn and send tension throughout the body, pushing a variety of metabolic symptoms off balance. As the hormone cortisol is released, your heart races and your hands get clammy, this is why a knot grows in your stomach and your chest tightens. Now, think about what you need to do today. How do you feel?

We all know how easy it is to turn on the stress systems. Turning them off, well that's something entirely different. As it turns out, it's very difficult to turn the brain on and off when it comes to stress. It's very difficult to manipulate molecule pathways that link the brain's infinitely complex network of 100 billion nerve cells, with virtually every other pathway, and to the tissues and organs in our body.

Threat, Pleasure and Novelty
I believe that if someone is hurting either physically or

emotionally, it is impossible to make good decisions for themselves or their loved ones.

There are basically two channels in our brain. One channel is activated when a person focuses on the external events or tasks like finishing a puzzle, appreciating a painting, or getting lost in a song. The other, brain channel is the product of internalizing thoughts, planning, thinking, and worrying. These internal thoughts are where the trouble lies.

Everything that competes for our attention falls into one of three categories: threat, pleasure or novelty. Early man looked at threat as a more mortal danger; like predators, floods and fires. Today, most of the threats we encounter are of our own making; such as: anxiety about an upcoming engagement, guilt over things we have done or haven't done, or fear of the future. Looking at these threats, it doesn't seem to pack the same punch, as a hungry lion would have on us; they both get our attention, none the same. When we put ourselves into this black hole of threat, we sink in and it is very difficult to free ourselves from its gravitational pull. Complicating our escape, is the fact that a stressful state often becomes the brain's default button setting to ON; it slips ON almost automatically. Blame human biology. Like a gym trained muscle, the plasticity of the brain allows frequently used nerves and networks to grow stronger. So, over time, familiar pathways become well-worn like a rut in a country road and our thoughts end up stuck, following routes that take them somewhere other than where we want them to go. Soon, our obsessing over perceived threats is our norm.

We go to bed with our head spinning and our body churning, and it's nobody's fault. It's ingrained in the way that these networks are set up. The stress response was always meant for emergencies, a quick and focused response to impeding and immediate disaster. But modern day stress, such as threats of, job: security, your failing 401(k), and your daughter's new questionable boyfriend, tend to linger. Neither our brain nor our body was designed to manage that kind of sustained stress. So the body protests and can rebels in a variety of forms, such as heart disease, hypertension, stroke, depression, and on and on.

Getting Off Stuck!
"The only disability in life is a bad attitude" Scott Hamilton

Fortunately, just as those well-worn negative pathways can be created, they also can be redirected. The key is learning to recognize what it feels like when your brain begins to slip into the default state. Only then can you work on breaking free of its grip. Eventually, what once took conscious effort to adjust, will become another circuit in the new default.

Rebuilding our mental infrastructure means being able to focus on the task or experience at hand. We just need to shut off any of our other distractions and thoughts. That's what meditation experts are advocating when they talk about emptying the mind or be in the moment. This is what they hope to accomplish when they ask clients to concentrate on their breathing.

Of course the more ingrained the stress pathways, the more difficult the seemingly uncomplicated tasks can be. You just have to train your brain on one thought at a time. Start with those very first thoughts in the morning. Don't think about the responsibilities of the day. Welcome the day, instead! Choose to think about what needs to be done, then be grateful that you know what is needed. Take five or ten minute breaks throughout the day by removing yourself from the pressures of the moment. Relax and be in gratitude. You can take a walk or change the scenery, sometimes that's all it takes. Choose to think about nothing, and if something comes to mind, let it float right back out. Just let yourself get away. It only takes five or ten minutes to get great results.

Balancing It All
I may embrace a health regimen based on science. Yet, I can do more than eat well, exercise and hope for the best. Wellness includes attention to my brain, body, mind, spirit and emotions.

Keeping our hormones balanced, keeps our brain more balanced and in turn keeps our body more balanced.

Meditation teaches us to fully engage in the moment, which calms the limbic system and increase activity in the higher cortical brain. There are pictures to support this in a 2005 study showing participants who meditated over long periods of time, had thicker cortices then those who didn't. A more recent study found improvement in the white matter of the subjects who had completed four weeks of integrated body/mind training.

Managing stress is important. Little stresses, every now and then in challenging situations, can push the brain to heighten competency. Chronic negative stress releases chemicals that inhibit neurogenesis and cause adverse physical changes in the brain.

An adult brain is not unchangeable, as it had long been believed. Rather, it is neural plastic; subject to physical modifications caused by life experiences and environmental factors. Scientists have proved that the adult brain is capable of neurogenesis, the process of creating new cells, even as it loses volume. Finally, while the brain often loses volume or size, in speed and efficiency as, believed in years past, there is a lot of variation in how much and how fast. Put this all together, and it spells serious hope for the aging brain. With possibilities, comes responsibility. Brains don't heal themselves.

For those of you who want help, science and technology offers the ageing, pharmaceuticals and supplements, even video games that promise to keep your aging brain savvy and sharp. But, not even the magic pill can counteract the effects of brain aging, if the person taking the pill engages in a lifestyle that accelerates the declining effects on the brain. If you eat organic food only, but still drink plenty of alcohol and smoke a pack of tobacco a day, what are you doing to your brain?

We all hope to continue good physical health as we age, yes, but what good is it if we don't have all of our marbles. At the very best, we want to know we won't end up staring at something or someone previously familiar to us and not be able to recognize or name them. What we think of as sharpness, the cognitive ability to choose a health plan, use a new cell phone, or understand a joke, is regulated in our cerebral cortex, the deeply wrinkled layer of gray matter on the outside of our brains. The older we get, the less cortex we have.

In a 2004 study, it was found that the thickness and the volume of the surface area of the cortex of a healthy individual, diminish with age. This shrinkage at age 30 is already showing signs of thinning and by 60 this reduction is profound. This is not the only damage to worry about, either. The aging brain loses not only gray matter, but also some of the white matter below it. Myelin is the insulating fatty material that coats the brain and its scarcity is implicated in many neurodegenerative diseases, including dementia and Alzheimer's, but also in healthy aging brains. The loss is believed to slow processing speeds and decrease the number of neutral connections. This explains why the elderly, on average, do worse on tasks that require paying attention to lots of stimuli at the same time. Like driving, and holding onto multiple pieces of information simultaneously planning a trip to a new destination. Relying on memory retrieval, such as remembering where the car was parked in a parking lot. Age related changes in the brain's topography are not the only threat. Consider inflammation, or our immune system response to injury. Chronic inflammation takes a toll on the aging body, causing cancer, heart disease, diabetes and cognitive problems. Similarly, the brain has been linked to various conditions, including depression, Alzheimer's and Parkinson's disease.

To keep our brain healthy, we need to keep learning, use novel intelligent tasks such as puzzle solving, learning a new instrument, learning a new language, and one of the best is dancing. All of these stimulate the brain to form new connections. Learning to juggle balls or pins, for example, has been shown to trigger at least short-term structural changes in the brain. Often brain training exercises primarily help people perform a particular task better. So doing the daily crossword puzzle will improve your crossword solving skills. But don't count on it to help you program the TV remote or any other new skill. It is important to learn NEW things every day. OK, I know you don't want to change or do something new. You say, you have always done it this way and you will continue doing it the same way. Or you may say "why reinvent the wheel?" It has been working just fine. You asked, why change? Without change we will get more of the same out of life. How is the "same" working in your life?

Make small changes. If you can start with something simple,

it is easier. Try brushing your teeth with your non- dominate hand. How did you do? Did you find that it was ridiculous to try something like that because your dominant hand has been doing it just fine? By using your non-dominant hand, just that one time, you woke up a different part of your brain and it was effortlessly done. When I try to do something just the opposite of what I normally do, I often laugh at myself. I was not as successful at brushing my teeth with my non-dominant hand. I got toothpaste all over the mirror and on the countertops. Obviously, it was messy. However, I know my brain is much happier and healthier because I did it. I even picture my brain putting on a happy face. Try laughing at yourself when you are not successful at something. Nobody but you saw you brushing your teeth with your non-dominant hand and making a mess. Lighten up and enjoy the journey.

You may not realize that you are creating the orders you need to give your brain today. However, this is precisely what you're doing. In this custom world that we live in, there needs to be a creator. The creator is not your brain (hard drive). IT'S YOU, your mind (soft ware). You need to be fully aware as creator, so the brain can do its best. You need to be the Leader for your brain as well as the inventor, teacher and user in order to have far more fulfilling results than what you have been achieving. As a leader, you make a decision such as, "I will have the same breakfast today as I had yesterday." As a better leader you can ask "What will I have for breakfast today that is different?" When you say "I want something new," then suddenly you are tapping into a reservoir of creativity. Creativity is a living, breathing new inspiration.

Ask the Brain

I love to see the flowers awaken to a new day. As the sunlight touches them, They respond by opening their petals in a beautiful display of color. In this same way, I open up my brain.

The brain has a miraculous ability to give more, when you ask more of it. You probably find that you don't ask much more today from your brain than you did the day before. But you can increase your brain activity by looking at each day in a new way. Pay attention not to fall into bad habits. Remind yourself that you can break this bad habit. Try improvising, ward off being bored, and gravitate to new things in many areas of your life. The word BORED is not part of my vocabulary. When I hear someone especially a child say, "I am bored" I instantly respond by giving them some tools and try to inspire them to take action not to be bored. Being bored is a learned bad habit. Of course this action may not make everyone happy when I do so.

Your brain is constantly evolving. This happens individually. The heart and the liver are essentially the same organs that you were born with, as they are when you die. Not your brain. It is capable of evolving and improving throughout your lifetime. Invent new things for your brain to do and you will become a source of new skills. I personally make bettering my brain an adventure. Like traveling to new places around the globe is an adventure..... so is my everyday life.

We live and learn a series of skills, beginning with walking, talking and reading. The mistake that we make is to limit our skills. Yet, at the same time, that sense of balance that allowed you to toddle, walk, run and then ride a bicycle is the balancing I am asking you to do with your brain, now. You are asking very little of your brain if you stop asking it to perfect a new skill every day. Ask yourself these questions. "Am I really saying my brain is growing just as much as when I was younger? If I try to learn a new skill, will I do the best I can? Sometimes, do I resent and resist change because I feel threatened by it? Why don't I reach beyond what I am really good at? Why don't I want to try it, even if it is just for fun? Do I spend too much time on passive things, like watching television?" What were your answers to these questions?

The brain wants more. Give your brain a good workout. Ask yourself these questions: "How can I adapt quickly to change? Can I remind myself that when I was a child, I first had to learn to walk before I could run? Find a way to make new challenges fun. I personally thrive on new activities.

Be the teacher of your brain. Knowledge is not rooted in facts, it is rooted in curiosity. Instilling curiosity is one's responsibility and at the same time you will feel inspired. No brain was ever inspired, but when your personality or ego is inspired you are triggering a cascade of reactions that light up the brain. There is evidence that we may prevent symptoms of senility and brain aging by remaining socially engaged and intellectually curious during our whole entire lifetime. Like a bright pupil, you must remain open to the things you don't know and be receptive rather than close minded to things you don't know.

In one study, people with difficult jobs, whether due to the work or the stress levels involved, were 80% less likely to age prematurely than those rare few enjoying an easy "dream job." Regularly having to face challenging tasks that demand self-discipline and perseverance, boosts the flow of oxygen and nutrient rich blood to the brain, keeping you youthful. Jobs can be anything from raising a family, to budgeting, car pooling, caring for family health, inside the home activities, as well as, working in a demanding job for pay, or volunteering in your community. That may have been the past work history of your life, so now what?

Ask yourself "Are you pretty settled in how you approach life? Are you webbed into your beliefs and opinions? Do you live your life for others? Do you enjoy thinking you are the expert? Do you rarely watch educational television or attend public lectures? Has it been a while since you felt really inspired? or do you like reinventing yourself? Have you recently changed a long held belief or an opinion? Is there at least one thing that you are really good at? Do you gravitate towards educational outlets on television or in your community? Are you inspired by your life on a day-to-day basis?"

Getting off that same old train!

One of the ways I get unstuck and get my brain stimulated is by volunteering for something new and different, or something I have not done for a long time. I may volunteer to help a family member or friend do a task I might have done many times before, but doing it for someone else stimulates my brain in many ways.

> *"The word "impossible" is not in my dictionary."*
>
> *Declared Napoleon Bonaparte*

Chapter 11

No Brain Owner's Manual

Start looking for your patterns in life. After the age of seven, everyone has developed life patterns, Those patterns will provide a road map to your life's work.

Just like a car, the brain needs fuel, repairs and proper management. But unlike a car, the brain has no "owner's manual." Food is not the only nutrient (fuel), for the brain, but physical and mental exercise as well. Alcohol and tobacco are toxic, so exposing the brain to them is improper management, or misuse, of the brain. Anger, fear, stress and depression are also kinds of misuse.

Stress shuts down the prefrontal cortex. This part, of the brain, is for correcting errors and assessing situations. That is why some people feel like they are going crazy in traffic jams. Traffic can be a routine stress. However, the rage, frustration and/or helplessness, that some drivers feel, could indicate that the prefrontal cortex has stopped overriding the primal impulses that it is responsible for controlling. Road rage, toxic memories and wounds of old traumas are bad habits that you can break. Feeling out of control, in some areas of your life, or suffering from addictions will create an unhealthy brain.

Ask yourself the following questions...

⇒ Are my stress levels too high, but I put up with them?
⇒ Do I worry about depression and am I depressed?

➤ Is my life going in a direction that I don't want it to go in?

➤ Are my thoughts obsessive, scary and make me anxious?

The above are all choices. To make changes, you can make statements, like this one: "I feel out of control, but I can avoid stressful situations by walking away and letting go. For an example:

I recently was in a store and in a hurry. An older woman, in her 70's, was walking in front of me with her adult daughter. The daughter was nagging her mother and telling her she was stupid and didn't know anything about what was good for her. Her mother was yelling back to her daughter saying that she only came to visit her once or twice a month. So, how could the daughter know what was good for her! All three of us arrived at the elevator at the same time. I had a choice to make – ride the elevator with them or wait for the next elevator. I chose to avoid a toxic situation by waiting for the next elevator. I am glad I did not ride that first elevator: I felt great!

Another statements you could use are, "I will try to be in a good mood." "Despite unexpected events, my life is headed in, the direction I want it to go." "I like the way my mind thinks." You can follow a path of growth, achievement, personal satisfaction and acquiring new skills. Without realizing it, this way of "talking to yourself" will make you capable of taking a quantum leap in how you use your brain. You will develop a relationship with your brain as you observe and become the silent witness to everything that your brain is doing.

Stay connected to friends and family. Make new friends. Making new friends requires the brain to perform mental tasks such as recognizing faces, recalling names, following conversations and producing appropriate responses. A good social life can provide a network of friends for your emotional support.

The brain is not a muscle, but it can benefit from a workout. Exercising the body increases the flow of blood, oxygen and nutrients and carries them to the brain. Also, physical exertion causes the release of a brain neurotrophic factor, which is a protein that bolsters existing neurons and encourages the growth of new ones. A healthy heart is a healthy brain. Every cell in the body needs a steady supply of oxygen and nutrients for the body to work properly. A healthy heart keeps those supply lines open. Anything that impedes blood flow, like high blood pressure or high cholesterol, will have a terrible effect on all organs including the brain. You can boost the brain power through diet by emphasizing choices that include antioxidants and inflammation fighters. If this brain wellness sounds familiar, it's because it is. The habits that will keep you sharp in later years are the same ones that will help you get to 100 years of age. A healthy heart diet, plus exercise is a diet and exercise for a healthy brain. So use your brain as much as possible. Do active cognitive tasks and maintain a vibrant social life. As we age, it is too easy to retire into solitude – just us and our TV. We need to keep working our brains. So get out there. GO!

The Pain's Message (that never fails!)

Pain, pain, go away! When the hurt lingers, physical pain and discomfort are only part of the problem. Erasing the emotional toll may offer the most relief. Pain is just a symptom, not a disease. While most of us know one can scrape a knee, cut a finger, or break a bone, the resulting pain is just alerting the body to the pathological process going on inside of us. Pain is an "it's an in-your-face" response!

Review Roberta's story in chapter three, as an example!

Pain is a message that never fails to attract our attention. Pain is about getting our attention. While pain is about attention and sensation, it is also about emotion. The emotional component, of course, evolution speaking, has been in existent since the Stone Age. Survival has often depended on pain being strong enough that we do whatever needs to be done or do whatever it takes to make it go away. The pain in my neck gets my attention, then that pain gives me a sensation and then my emotions kick in. All of these factors are the foundation for the kind of "web" located in the brain. This webbing connects parts of the brain that detect signals with those that respond emotionally via chemical messengers called neurotransmitters. Break some of the web threads and distract those messengers and you can free yourself from its clutches. Maybe the underlining pathology will still be there, but it will no longer be a pain in my neck.

Scientists call this the pain matrix. You bend over to pick up a large box of books but forget the old advice to lift with your legs. Before you are fully straightened up, do you detect trouble? Part of that realization comes from the actual sensation that you recognize, instantly, when the hyperactive cortex, the piece of the brain that receives and interprets the nerve signals, rise up your spine. When you felt that first flinch, you regarded it with something other than a chemical call. Your stomach was caught in your throat. You yelled, maybe even cried. In short you responded emotionally. Acute pain knows how to get your attention. Any late strong feelings, both emotionally and physically, show up. Brain imaging studies can actually show a pain signal, when it gets activated in the prefrontal cortex and in the anterior cortex. These two important areas, of the brain, provide emotional color to the pain experience in the scan. The scan shows the brain focusing on the pain, by lighting up the brain's emotional centers. Normally, these components of the brain matrix are in balance. Stub your toe and you hop up and down in pain or screaming in anger. Within minutes, the throbbing begins to subside and with it, go your emotions. Sometimes however, the pain doesn't go away. Faced with an increasing barrage, of pain signals, the brain falls a bit out of sync. Because it can only surmise that its neurochemical distress calls are going unheeded, it yells louder. At some point, the emotional components of the pain become the predominant signals. Feeding on itself, the sensation of pain can end up lasting long after the actual pain stimulants, are gone or reduced. Chronic pain, by definition, is hard to solve. When conventional medicine falls short, complementary therapies often get the call. You're not likely to run to an acupuncturist or a massage therapist for a stubbed toe. However, for a migraine headache, that won't quit, you will do anything to silence it. At their core, most integrative pain reducing techniques try to get the brain to shift attention from the chemicals like cortisol, to the ones that make you feel less stressed, such as serotonin or norepinephrine. These chemicals tend to make one feel happier and/or calmer.

How Hormones Help With Healing!

Reminiscing about the good times you once had
triggers your calming hormone to kick in
"Serotonin."

Create a bucket list of activities, then do some of
them, you kick in your pleasure hormone
"Dopamine."

Look into a mirror and do some power poses
for just 2 minutes kicks in your
"Testosterone."

Tap into your support system by cuddling. Research
has found that there are 58 different cuddling positions.
This creates a feeling of warmth and kicks in your
"Oxytocin."

Moving the body kicks in your
"Endorphin."
Endorphin hormones respond to pain in a natural way by
blocking your pain receptors. This may be one reason why we
sometimes do not feel acute pain immediately after an injury.

Spine Chart

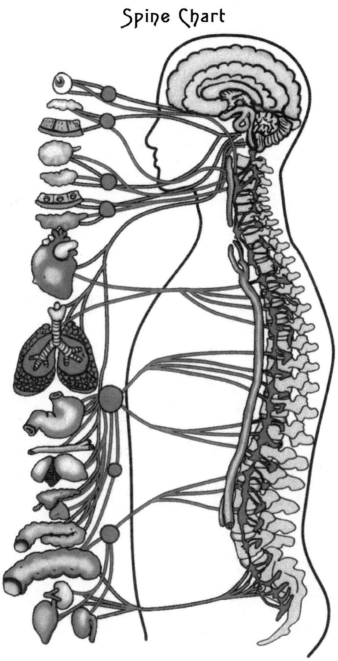

Having difficulty with one of your vertebras?
How is that vertebra affecting your body?

Chapter 12

Possibility Thinking

"Some men see things as they are and say 'Why'?" "I dream of things that never were and say 'Why not'?" John F. Kennedy popularized this George Bernard Shaw's stirring statement.

S o my question to myself is: Am I unleashing the enthusiasm of possibility- thinking in my life to find solutions for even the seemingly impossible situations? Can you ask yourself that question? People who believe they can't, won't. But if you believe in yourself, have confidence in your ability and have faith and believe you can, then you can! You have power within yourself, but don't be afraid to ask for help. Tell your story.

I believe that we can change our health no matter how old we are. I have seen many do it. We can make a difference by starting now.

Neurological Stress

What is neurological stress? The human body can respond and adapt to just about anything it encounters, provided it is in a state of homeostasis; which means that the body is able to send and receive nerve information. The central nervous system is the master control system of the body and every single function reflects its activity. Nerve impulses travel from the brain down the spinal cord and out through the nerves to all parts of the body. Nerve impulses then return to the brain via the spinal cord and up to the brain. There is an excess of 100 billion neurons, and nerve cells in the human central nervous system. The number of possible interconnections between the cells is greater than the total number of electrons in the known universe.

Now talking about the health of the central nervous system, we must talk a little about the skeletal support system. The spinal cord is encased by the spinal column which is made up of vertebrae. The tinniest and most delicate bones of the spine are those of the neck which are called cervical vertebrae, seven in all. Yet in spite of their size, the cervical vertebrae have the huge job of supporting the head, protecting the spinal cord, and providing mobility of the head and neck.

The top two cervical vertebrae are the most important: C1, the Atlas, is what the head rests on and C2, the Axis, is what rotates the head. The brainstem connects to the Atlas and Axis through an opening at the base of the skull. The job of the Atlas and Axis in essence is to protect the delicate brainstem without causing interference. The brainstem houses all control centers; messaging between the brain and the rest of the body; such as our basic body functions: breathing, swallowing, heart rate, blood pressure, consciousness, cardiac and respiratory functions and acts as a vehicle for sensory response and whether one is awake or a sleep. It is one of the most vital regions of our body. You can see how important the brainstem is and how essential it is to protect.

When the spine is straight, your head weighs about 10-14 pounds; much like a bowling ball. When you lean your neck and head forward just 15 degrees your head becomes a 27 pound weight. If you bend over; like when you are texting, cooking or writing, it becomes more like the weight of an eight-year-old sitting on your head.

It is very important to stand upright. As we age, the use of canes and walkers become a problem for our brainstem which affects our brain and body in so many ways. The best way to train the body to stand upright is to go to a market where they have grocery carts. When using a cart, you can't look down but rather you are forced to look at the horizon. Not only is it good exercise for the body, but pushing around a grocery cart keeps the spine straight, which gives the nerves an opportunity to communicate correctly to the bran by affecting this area, you can affect every area in your body, for good or for bad, in sickness or in health. It is your choice.

As I mentioned earlier, the nerve impulse travel from the brain down the spinal cord and out through the nerves to organs and the rest of the body. Where the nerves actually come out from the spine is, in between the vertebrae. One way problems can arise, is when the vertebrae are misaligned, which then impede the flow of information along the nerves to destination causing pain or disease.

The spine and nerve chart in this book, gives the different vertebrae and nerve correlating to an organ or body area they are responsible for. Using this chart, you can analyze which nerve is giving you problems. Then by using modalities such as chiropractic, acupuncture, massage or physical therapy or something as simple as pushing a shopping cart around, one may alleviate pinched nerves and keep the body in alignment. By keeping the body in alignment the muscles and tendons will help support the alignment and this maintains a more balanced brain. A balanced brain means a healthier body!

Talking about neurological stress and how under optimal conditions the body can respond and adapt to anything it encounters, provided that the body is able to send and receive nerve information. When under stress, our brain perceives a threat to our wellbeing. Adrenaline shoots out from our adrenal glands virtually instantaneously. It is the only gland that has a direct nerve connection from the spinal cord. This allows it to give and instant response when lifesaving action has to be taken immediately. It does not wait around for the cortisol to be released into the bloodstream. When your body is in survival mode, it shuts down anything that is not essential for survival.

Here are a few ways our body processes shut down:

1. Immune system. You do not need to worry about viruses or bacteria if you are about to be eaten by a tiger. You must survive or escape the tiger first.
2. Digestive system. You don't need to be digesting the food you are eating if you are trying to avoid a bus coming right at you.

3. Short-term memory. It is totally useless and inappropriate in a sudden survival situation. You do not need to remember your grocery list right now.
4. Sex gland function. Once again, you have to survive the situation first or reproduction is a mute issue.
5. Logical thinking. Too slow. You need to respond instinctively. You're not going to think "well, he looks like an old tiger without any teeth." You are not going to think logically.
6. Relaxation and pleasure. Totally inappropriate response to "I might get eaten by this tiger!" STRESS AND ANXIETY GOES UP.
7. Muscle relaxation. You don't need your muscles to relax; you need them on high alert.

What does this have to do with your day to day life? EVERYTHING.

Our entire body is wired for cell signaling so that the body can repair, restore and/or coordinate physiological and psychological activities.

To stay healthy as well as repair the cell damage during aging, our cells continuously talk to each other to know how to behave in relationship to the surrounding environment. Cell signaling or cell communication, is fundamental to coping with stress; the underlying component of functional aging. Aging can be defined as a gradual loss of the ability to respond or adapt to its environment. Recent studies have provided evidence that, indeed our brain may control our life span. We may not be able to control our generic factors; however, we can certainly change the way we respond to our environment by being in control of our brain and body. Let us be good a steward.

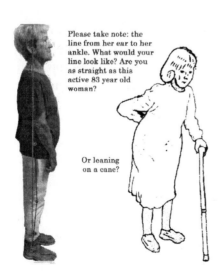

Please take note: the line from her ear to her ankle. What would your line look like? Are you as straight as this active 83 year old woman?

Or leaning on a cane?

Chapter 13

"I Think I Can"

John Andrew Holmes said "Never tell a young person that something cannot be done. God may have been waiting centuries for somebody unknowing enough, of the impossible, to do that thing."

Personally, I have learned to use the word impossible with the greatest of caution. If you want to achieve something, give yourself permission to believe it is possible, no matter what experts say. That was what I did when doctors said. "You will never get better." They also said. "You will never be able to take care of yourself again." Another doctor said. "Linda, you will need others to always take care your basic needs."

Sure it has been hard work, and still is, but I continue working on my brain and body every day. All in all, I try and balance every aspect of my life each and every day. Am I successful all the time? NO, but when I fail one day, I start all over the next day and keep at it. I am like the "Little Engine That Could." I say to myself "I think I can, I think I can, I think I can!" And pretty soon I do.

I can't believe how many times people have told me they have never had a concussion, hit their head or been hit in the head. Other times, people will describe their auto accident they got a broken nose, a broken collar bone, plus all their cuts and bruises. All the while, failing to tell me that they rolled over and over down a "100" foot embankment and landed upside down. In summary they didn't have a head injury, because they had their seatbelt on. Oh yes, and then they were rushed to the hospital and treated just for their broken bones, cuts and bruises. Only in recent years have head injuries and TBI's been included in exams after an accident. Doctors are beginning to understand about TBI's. In the coming years, there will be more research on brain injuries and TBI's.

TBI Traumatic Brain Injury

People with a TBI (traumatic brain injury), are not just football players or our military. A TBI can happen to anyone, at any age, and by many different causes. It could have happened years ago, but went undetected, that TBI may be causing brain issues today. Often times, there are accumulative injuries that cause problems.

I have worked with hundreds of clients with traumatic brain injuries. These are some characteristics of a traumatic brain injury: An injury caused by external trauma to the head or violent movement of the head, such as from a fall, blast, car crash or being shaken. TBI may or may not be combined with loss of consciousness, an open wound or skull fracture.

The purpose of including this information in the book is to inform readers that a TBI is a common problem. People with TBI may have difficulty with: impairments in memory, judgment, concentration, head pain, organization, task initiation and completion, among other things. Consequently, they may be unable to hold a job, live independently, or accomplish tasks of daily living. Many people with TBI might be undiagnosed. In order to evaluate service eligibility and make the appropriate referrals, the source of disability must be identified.

Who should be screened?

A person with a known trauma that could have caused a brain injury or a person having difficulty functioning or exhibiting unexplained behaviors

This TBI screening tool is a first step towards identifying and properly diagnosing a TBI.

The following questions are asked of those who may have a TBI:
   •   Have you ever hit your head or been hit on the head?

Think about all accidents that may have occurred to them at any age, even those that did not seem serious, such as vehicle accidents, falls, assaults, abuse, near a blast that rung your chimes, domestic violence and child abuse and also for military related injuries. A TBI can also occur from violent shaking of the head, such as being shaken as a baby or child.

Was the person ever seen in the emergency room, hospital or by a doctor because of an injury to the head?

Did the person ever lose consciousness or experience a period of being dazed and confused because of an injury to the head?

Circle all problems that have occurred since the injury:
- Headaches
- Dizziness
- Balance difficulties
- Vision changes & perceptual difficulties
- Low tolerance to light and noise
- Diminished tolerance to cognitive simulation
- Slowed processing speed
- Anxiety, depression
- Difficulty concentrating
- Difficulty remembering
- Difficulty reading, writing, calculating
- Poor planning
- Poor organizing
- Poor problem solving
- Poor goal director behavior
- Poor time management
- Poor quality management
- Changes in relationships
- Difficulty performing job or school work
- Diminished attention
- Increased distractibility
- Poor judgment; fights, fired from job or arrested
- Reduced awareness
- Low frustration
- Reduced impulse control
- Heightened anger and irritability
- Altered family role
- Unable to self monitor and regulate behavior

- Unsafe to operate motor vehicle
- Inability or tolerance to work demands
- Emotional adjustment & coping difficulties
- Reduced stamina
- Inability to participate in full range of pre-injury activities

Seeing marked changes in home or social activities, people with a TBI may not lose consciousness but experience an alteration of consciousness. This may include feeling dazed, confused or disoriented at the time of the injury or being unable to remember the events around the head injury.

Does the person experience any of these problems in daily life since the head injury? Is there any significant sickness? Note: Some of these symptoms could be a sign of a medical condition such as a brain tumor, meningitis, West Nile virus, stroke, seizures or oxygen deprivation such as a heart attack, carbon monoxide poising, near drowning or suffocation.

PTSD Post-traumatic stress disorder

What is PTSD; Post-traumatic stress disorder? Triggered by a terrifying event; either by experiencing it or witnessing it. Symptoms may include flashbacks, nightmares and severe anxiety, making it difficult to function through life. It is important to get effective treatment. PTSD may start within months or may not appear until years later. These symptoms (four types) cause significant problems with social interactions, work situations and in personal relationships.

1. **Intrusive:** Recurrent, unwanted distressing memories of the event, reliving the event as flashbacks, upsetting dreams about the event, severe emotional distress or physical reaction to something that reminds one of the event.
2. **Avoidance:** Trying to avoid thinking or talking about the event, avoiding places, activities or people that remind one of the event.
3. **Negative changes in thinking and mood:** Negative feelings about self or other people, inability to experience

positive emotions, feeling emotionally numb, lack of interest in an activity that was once enjoyed, hopelessness about the future, memory problems, not remembering important aspects of the event, difficulty maintaining close relationships.

4. **Changes in emotional reactions:** Irritability angry out bursts or aggressive behavior, always being on guard for danger, overwhelming guilt or shame, self destructive behavior like drinking too much or driving too fast, trouble concentrating, trouble sleeping, being easily startled or frightened.

PTSD could be caused by the severity of an event, or be a repeat of several events. Women are more likely to have PTSD than men. It is estimated one in ten women have PTSD.

It is very possible that a person can have a TBI and PTSD at the same time, as we have seen repeatedly in our veterans. One does not have to be a veteran to have both at once. It is determined by the event and the severity of that event. Be kind to your brain and be kind to those who have TBI and or PTSD. With patience and work your brain can get better.

Ylang Ylang
Uplifting and hikes happiness. This tropical flower lowers the heart rate and blood pressure. It triggers and floods the body with endorphins.

Jasmine
Enhances dexterity and eye hand coordination. Help those who are struggle with their handwriting, sewing or hitting a golf ball or baseball.

Chapter 14

Teeth and Hair Toxicity

No one can ever overcome anything until his thoughts are creative and positive.

Teeth Toxicity

E very tooth, in our mouth, is connected to a different part of our body. As we all know it is very important to take good care of our teeth. However, there is more to it. Mercury amalgam (silver) fillings are hazards to our health. Today, it's even more important to know the difference between a mercury free and mercury safe dentist. More and more dentists no longer use mercury amalgam fillings, because simply isn't as good compared to the newer composites. Increasingly, these dentists refer to their practice as being "mercury free." However, that doesn't mean that they believe that mercury fillings are a health hazard or that they will protect you from excessive exposure to mercury during the removal. Bottom line, a dentist who advertises mercury free composites, may not have the knowledge to safely remove mercury amalgam (silver).

Being protected during the amalgam removal is extremely important because the greatest exposure to mercury vapor occurs when the filling is unsafely removed. When the dentist uses the safe removal, the exposure to mercury amalgam is reduced by 90%. When unsafe drilling takes place to take out a mercury amalgam filling, it can release up to 4,000 mcg of mercury vapor.

The following list about mercury amalgam contains well established facts found in scientific literature.

1. There is no level of mercury exposure that is regarded as safe or harmless.
2. Originally placed silver amalgam fillings contain approximately 50% mercury.
3. Mercury is not locked in the fillings, so it does escape in small amounts, mostly in the form of volatilized mercury vapor.
4. Exposure to mercury increases with chewing, tooth brushing and heat.
5. Mercury vapor is extremely toxic and easily absorbed. Its toxicity is rated greater than lead, cadmium or arsenic.
6. Leading toxicologist has concluded that mercury, from amalgam fillings, constitutes the single greatest source of mercury exposure to humans. The toxic effect of mercury is greater than food, air or environmental toxicity to humans.
7. Animal studies have shown that amalgam derived mercury accumulates in body tissue and organs. It also travels through fetal blood and tissue and is found in maternal milk.

Tooth / Organ Relationship Chart

Left Side

Right Side

Glands	Anterior Pituitary	RIGHT BREAST Parathyroid	Thyroid	Thymus	Posterior Pituitary	Intermediate lobe of pituitary	Pineal	Pineal	Pineal	Intermediate lobe of pituitary	Posterior Pituitary	Thymus	Thyroid	LEFT BREAST Parathyroid	Anterior Pituitary
Organs	Heart / Small Intestines / Endocrine gland, Pericardial	Breast / Thyroid / Stomach / Pancreas		Lungs / Large Intestines		Liver / Gall Bladder / Eye	Kidneys / Prostate / Bladder, Uterus, Rectum, Anus			Liver / Gall Bladder / Eye		Lungs / Large Intestines		Breast / Thyroid / Stomach / Spleen	Heart / Small Intestines / Endocrine gland, Pericardial
Teeth	1	2	3	4	5	6	7	8	9	10	11	12	13	14	15	16
Upper Jaw	3rd Molar (wisdom)	2nd Molar	1st Molar	2nd Bicuspid (pre-molar)	1st Bicuspid (pre-molar)	Canine (cuspid)	Lateral incisor	Central incisor	Central incisor	Lateral incisor	Canine (cuspid)	1st Bicuspid (pre-molar)	2nd Bicuspid (pre-molar)	1st Molar	2nd Molar	3rd Molar (wisdom)
Lower Jaw	3rd Molar (wisdom)	2nd Molar	1st Molar	2nd Bicuspid (pre-molar)	1st Bicuspid (pre-molar)	Canine (cuspid)	Lateral incisor	Central incisor	Central incisor	Lateral incisor	Canine (cuspid)	1st Bicuspid (pre-molar)	2nd Bicuspid (pre-molar)	1st Molar	2nd Molar	3rd Molar (wisdom)
Teeth	32	31	30	29	28	27	26	25	24	23	22	21	20	19	18	17
Organs	Heart / Small Intestines / Endocrine gland, Pericardial	Lungs / Large Intestines		Stomach / Pancreas		Liver / Eye	Kidneys / Prostate / Bladder, Uterus, Rectum, Anus			Liver / Eye		Stomach / Spleen		Lungs / Large Intestines	Heart / Small Intestines / Endocrine gland, Pericardial
Glands	Fire	RIGHT BREAST	Earth	Ovaries / Metal	Metal	Testicles / Wood	Wood	Adrenals / Water	Water	Adrenals / Water	Ovaries / Wood	Testicles / Metal	LEFT BREAST	Earth	Fire
Element	Fire	Earth		Metal		Wood	Water			Water	Wood	Metal		Earth	Fire

85

Hair Toxicity

You probably heard of all different types of detoxify programs for your body, but did you know that you can also detoxify your hair? Detoxifying your scalp every once in awhile will help make your scalp healthy so your hair will be luscious and shiny. Hair detoxifying gets rid of chemicals, toxins and pollutants in your body, which are all bad for your health and your immune system. These toxins can make their way to your scalp and cause a number of common hair problems such as dandruff, dry hair, and split ends and hair loss. Harmful toxins to your hair and scalp include: Paradens, PEG-3 cocamide, diamine toluene sulfate and sodium lauryl/laureth sulfate. All of these toxins are in common shampoos, conditioners and other hair products.

Your hair is a living and breathing extension of your body, and your scalp contains some of the largest pores on your skin. To make sure that your hair is healthy, a routine regime of deep cleansing and purification is essential to creating a complete wellness program. After all, why would you detoxify your body, but keep putting toxins in your hair? An excellent way to draw out toxins on your scalp and to boost your immunity is to use a deep cleansing treatment that is free of parabens, PEG-3 cocamide, diamine toluene sulfate and sodium laury/laureth sulfate. A gentle, yet effective treatment; will lift heavy metals and other toxins from the hair follicles, scalp and oil glands, so your scalp is fresh and clean. This treatment helps promote hair growth and will leave your hair feeling clean and naturally healthy. Hair loss is common as we age, due to many factors, but using toxic substances on our hair and scalp should not be a factor in hair loss. Medication, diet, lack of blood flow along with illness and disease, are other possible factors.

I am ready to release burdens of anger, pain and shame. I forgive when I believe there is a better way. I am ready to experience freedom and love without limits. Also, I know that breaking out of familiar patterns takes great energy. I am ready!

Sandalwood
Stimulates receptors in your skin that signal skin cells to regenerate faster, improving healing and creating newer younger skin.

Myrrh
This relaxing aroma stimulates the production of soothing brain waves, ending edginess and blah moods and can be used in tea form.

Chapter 15

Fibromyalgia! The Different Kinds

Henry Ford said:
"Failure is the opportunity to begin again, more intelligently"

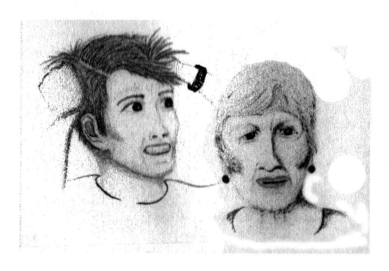

Are you confused? Or know someone who is?

To get a better understanding of fibromyalgia and the symptoms read the following:

Cerebral: fatigue, irritability, nervousness, depression, impaired memory and concentration, apathy, frequent awakening during the night, non-restored sleep, blurred vision, dizziness and headaches, often called migraines.

Musculoskeletal: widespread throughout the body, aching pain and stiffness in the muscles, tendons and ligaments, in the morning which are often worse. Pain can assume any form and intensity, such as throbbing, burning, stabbing, stinging and grabbing or any combination of these pain symptoms. Numbness showing up in the arms, hands, feet, legs, or face and tingling anywhere in the body, usually from contracted structures pressing on nearby nerves.

TMJ: jaw joint pain, possibly with difficulty chewing, and excruciating pain in the face and head, originating in the neck. Muscles can often be seen twitching anywhere in the body and the restless leg syndrome can make it impossible to find a comfortable spot. Sometimes it feels like electrical impulses in the muscles and a feeling of general weakness.

Dermal: a creepy crawly feeling, itching, many varieties of rashes, burning and sometimes swollen, hot itchy palms or soles of the feet. Signs of patchy pimples and perspiration are both pungent and irritating the skin.

Gastrointestinal: Known as "Fibro gut," it's an irritable bowel syndrome that includes gas, pain, bloating, constipation alternating with diarrhea, and may cause nausea or hyperacidity.

Genitourinary: Vulvodynia which includes raw, irritated, burning vaginal lips and vulva pain, vaginal spasm and cramps, burning discharge, increased menstrual and uterine cramps, painful intercourse, repeated bladder infections, pungent, concentrated urine, and chronic interstitial cysts.

Miscellaneous: Excessive nasal congestion and mucus, brittle nails, inferior hair quality, hair dryness, signs of dry, scalded or metallic mouth sensations. Eye irritation or burning with discharge or burning tears, and may have transient ringing in the ears. Dizziness and true vertigo arises in the middle ear which often is a complaint of increase sensitivity to sound, bright lights, smells and sensitivity to certain chemicals.

The broad spectrum of body functions and tissue affected by fibromyalgia are chronic fatigue, chronic Candida, and bulbar pain, along with myofascial pain syndrome are all names for the same fibromyalgia disease. Over time, the accumulation progresses within more and more cells, resulting in an energy deficiency, are starting with a certain system, but eventually running throughout the body. At this time, the disease makes itself known. You will find that every function of the body needs energy, not only to move, run, exercise, and speak, but also simply to grow hair, breed, digest food, beat illness, and especially to use our brains. Our cells use a current of energy known as a biochemical term, ATP, to perform metabolic chores and other crucial tasks that are vital to our existence. Improperly functioning cells and the concentration of phosphate and other substances are integral to energy formation is meticulously maintained.

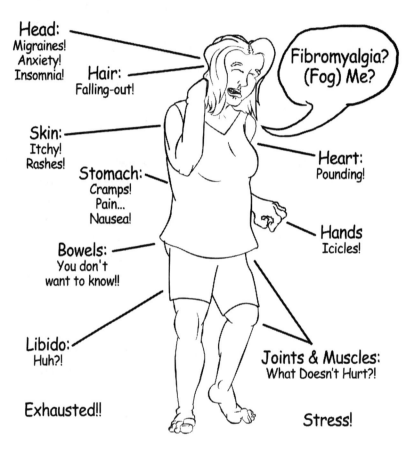

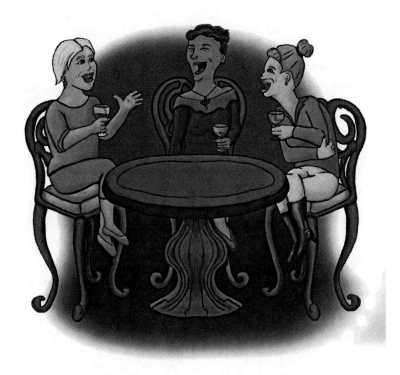

How does it seem that you always get your way?
Oh, Honey I whine a lot.

Have a real conversation by engaging
with five people living outside
your home everyday. No social media,
use phone calls or face to face
engaging conversations.

Chapter 16

Super Brain Yoga

"You may prefer to be content to go forth alone, yet with others you go farther and faster. One wall standing alone is useless yet should one put three or four walls together they will support a roof and keep the grain dry." ~ By Rumi

Super Brain Yoga, created by Master Choa Kok Sui.
I use Super Brain Yoga when I am hurting, either physically or emotionally, instead of taking any medication. If I wake up in the middle of the night and have trouble going back to sleep, I use Super Brain Yoga. I use it when I have cognitive problems, balance problems or having trouble just remembering everyday things. For any of the above conditions, I usually get relief within 20 to 30 minutes.

Twenty percent of the body's total energy expenditure is consumed by the brain. The average person can store up to 1 million items in the brain. A scientific breakthrough has demonstrated conclusively that the human brain can give rise to new brain cells and spawn new neurons to regenerate it and repair broken circuitry's caused by aging, damage or disease. Neural plasticity of the brain's ability to recognize neural pathways can be benefited by doing Super Brain Yoga.

In recent years, researchers have found that exercise improves memory, concentration, and abstract reasoning among older adults, super brain yoga works like this; aerobic exercise increases the blood flow to the brain, which nurses brain cells and allows them to function more effectively. It's kind of like making sure your engine is all tuned up. A recent study showed that exercise can actually promote the growth of new neurons and brain cells in the hippocampus, the part of the brain that controls memory and learning. Scientists previously believed that once the brain cells die, they were not replaced. You can get cognitive benefits with activity that is fairly simple, like walking for 20 minutes a day or using Super Brain Yoga. While yoga has long been shown to affect mood, one yoga move in particular is getting attention for boosting brainpower. "Super Brain Yoga," as the exercise is called, is being participated in across the country as an antidote to brain drain. Go ahead and try it. The simple moves boost brain function by stimulating acupuncture points on the earlobes. By doing this yoga exercise you are improving both the physical body and the energy body. A lot of sickness is caused in part by the malfunctioning of one or more of our energy centers.

Acupuncture points are made up of two parts, an upper part and the lower part. These two parts are consistently moving in opposite directions. When the upper part is moving clockwise, the lower part is moving counterclockwise. This motion alternates from clockwise to counterclockwise. The body is like a complicated electronic piece of equipment. When the proper energy wiring connection is made, it produces the right results. When the connection is wrong, it does not produce the expected results. The right earlobe corresponds with the left brain, while the left earlobe corresponds with the right brain. The right earlobe is gently squeezed with the left thumb and left index finger, with the thumb on the outside. It produces the necessary energy connection which causes left brain and pituitary gland to become energized and activated. When the left earlobe is gently squeezed with the right thumb and right index finger with the thumb on the outside, it produces the necessary energy connection which causes the right brain pineal gland to become energized and activated. If you use the right thumb and index finger to gently squeeze the right earlobe this exercise will not work, because it's the wrong hand and will not connect to the brain correctly. Also, if you use the left thumb and index finger to gently squeeze the left earlobe it also will not work, because you are using the wrong hand. Also, the right arm must be outside while the left arm must be inside by doing so this will increase the brain to become energized and activated. The arms are crossing over the chest. Do Super Brain Yoga standing up.

There are a few words of caution when doing this exercise, keep a chair within arm's length and use it if you get out of balance in any way. As a precaution, if you're pregnant do not use this exercise because there are no known studies of these exercises and pregnancy.

If you are having trouble with any part of the Super Brain Yoga exercises, is just an indication that particular part of your brain needs to be activated and healed. Don't give up, in time it will become easier and easier for you to accomplish the successes that Super Brain Yoga has to offer. You may find that once a day is all you'll need to get the results that you want to obtain.

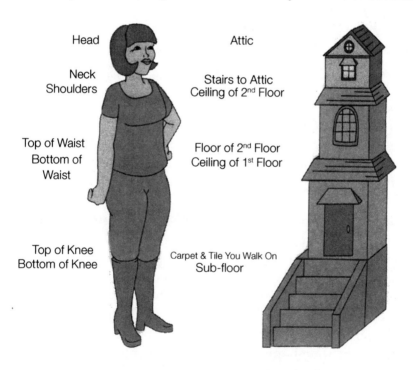

Think of your body as a three story house.
Compare these two for a better understanding
of your body.

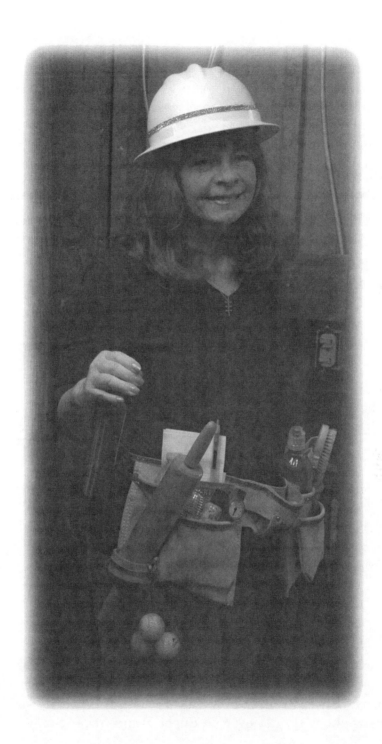

Chapter 17

Techniques and Tools

"Let no one come to you without ever leaving better and happier. Be the living expression of God's kindness: kindness in your face, And kindness in your eyes, and kindness in your smile."
~ Mother Teresa quote

The information in this book may not apply to all people with the same issues, each person may respond differently. We may all have two eyes, two arms and two feet, but there are no two bodies alike.

Advice to Readers; Before following any techniques contained in this book, it is recommended that you consult your doctor or your health care professionals. If you suffer from any health problems, have special conditions, or are in doubt, as to its suitability towards these techniques and your health, consult the appropriate professional.

⇒⟫ • ⟪⇐

Technique
SUPERBRAIN YOGA
by Grand Master Choa Kok Sui

As a precaution, if you're pregnant do not use this exercise, because there are no known studies of the exercises and pregnancy. Do not do Super Brain Yoga two days before, during and two after menstruation. Do not over do Super Brain Yoga it may cause insomnia, or weakening of the body, pain or discomfort or skin rashes. It is recommended not to do more than once a day.

Place Your Tongue to the Roof of Mouth
Stand, facing east, for the ill and elderly face north

Exercises:

Always start with the right side and go to the right first... Stand and line up hips up with shoulders... All exercise will be done to a count of 12, except #9 and #11... If you can, take a breath in when initiating pose, then blow out to move.

1. Place your right hand in front of your eyes away from your face. Watch your hand turn to the right, in a circle, 12 times. Repeat with the left hand turning to the left 12 times.
2. Turn your head from right to left 12 times. (R1, L1, R2, L2, and so on) 12 times.
3. Drop your chin to the chest and blow out as your chin drops. 12 times.
4. Reach up to the sky with your right arm up overhead, then repeat lifting left arm overhead. R1, L1, R2, L2, 12 times
5. Twist your upper body to the right and then to the left. R1, L1, R2, L2 12 times.
6. Roll your shoulders and arms forward, 12 times. Roll your shoulders and arms backwards 12 times.
7. Place your hands on hips and move your hips as if you are using a hula hoop to the right 12 times and then to the left 12 times.
8. Do short fast squats, like riding a horse (50 times). Breath in when going down and breath out when coming up.
9. Place your hands on both knees and circle knees to the right 12 times and then to the left 12 times.
10. While standing, circle right foot to right at the ankle 12 times and then circle right foot to the left, then point the right foot up and down 12 times. Repeat each with left foot 12 times. Hold on to a chair if needed to keep your balance.

11. Place your left thumb on right ear with thumb facing forward of ear and your index finger on back of right ear. Then place your right thumb on left ear, crossing right arm over left arm, thumb facing forward and your index finger on back of left ear. Slowly breathe in as you squat down, then again slowly breathe out as you stand up. Repeat 14 times.

⇒≫ • ≪⇐

Technique

HOW THE MOON AFFECTS US
~ *Mark it on the calendar* ~

Our body has the same percent of water that the earth dose. The moon creates waves and causes turbulence in the ocean and it also causes turbulence in our body. Our brain, separate from our body, has the same percentage of water ratio as the earth. When the full moon comes out, it creates havoc on our body and brain. Just talk to any ER doctor or policeman and they will tell you how difficult their job is during the full moon.

I have found that when we are young and healthy that two days before the full moon, and the day of the full moon, and two days after the full moon people have a hard time sleeping and don't feel up to par. These same people could also be affected by the new moon. This time period is the day before, the day of, and the day after the new moon. However, for the elderly, three days before the new moon, the day of the new moon and three days after the new moon. The elderly are affected by the full moon four days before, the day of, and four days after the full moon.

I have also found that if a young child is very sick, or an elderly person is very sick they might need to add an extra day on each end of the full moon and new moon. Keep track of this on a calendar and you will discover your patterns. There have been many studies on this subject in this country and other countries. Solar flares and meteor showers; can also affect our sleep and keep us feeling not up to par.

*"Don't die before your death" or you are just wasting your
life while waiting to die? Don't die, start living!"*

⇛ • ⇚

Write a full page of "I WANT." This could be a "bucket list."
Write ways to live a better life or have better health. This list
is whatever you want to write. We need to get into the habit of
saying what we want. The "I want" are not only for ourselves, but
to better communicate with others. We need to speak as naturally,
as possible when we are communicating. Don't just think about
them, write them down. When writing them down, make a note
of how you feel. Ask yourself questions: what am I thinking? Am
I smiling about what I am writing about? Do I feel uncomfortable?
Do I feel special? Get to know yourself. When you get to know
yourself, others will get to know you better. You may find that life
is much easier and fulfilling.

⇛ • ⇚

Technique
BE GRATIFULL!
Write down your gratitudes

Write 5 gratitudes per day. As you write down your gratitude
include all your senses. Really put your whole body into feeling
the gratitude as you are writing. They can be as simple as noticing
someone letting you go first when you are driving. It can be as
big as winning the Lotto or moving out of state. Do these each
day, any time of the day. Just notice as they happen. Take note
how you feel what you are thinking. Are you smiling? Do you
feel uncomfortable? Do you feel special? Do you think you are
lucky? Some people feel uncomfortable when they are receiving
something or got lucky. When I was unable to remember in the
evening, what I did in that morning, I had to write my gratitude
down in my notebook, right then and there, or I had nothing to

show for the day. I would look at my gratitude list often, as it encouraged me to continue moving forward. I am now grateful for the energy and strength of my healthier body.

⇛ • ⇚

Technique
GIVE FROM THE HEART ANONYMOUSLY!

I can't tell you how many times I have heard "I give all the time" or "It is stupid to give without letting them know I gave it to them." How do you like this one- "Charity starts at home." You may be right, but I can tell you, if you do this giving anonymously, your life will become more balanced and much richer. Each day, give from the heart anonymously without expecting anything in return. It can for example, be something like opening the door for someone. You could help a woman with her packages, while she is trying to care for her kids. Take the trash cans out for a sick neighbor, so the trash truck can pick them up. It can be something as simple as buying a stranger a movie ticket that the cashier gives to someone further back in line. Try doing something nice when you're late to your destination, like let someone go in front of you. Try paying it forward. Take note how you feel: what you are thinking, are you smiling, do you feel uncomfortable, do you feel special, do you think that person was lucky you came along or do you think you are lucky?

When you are doing the above; (I want, Gratitude and Giving from the Heart Anonymously) you are giving your body's cellular memory a chance to change and heal. People tell me the hardest one to do is; "Give from the Heart Anonymously" and not expect anything in return. Next hardest to do is "I want." The more you do these, the easier it gets.

The cellular memory can be healed!
Most cells of the body rejuvenate themselves and are completely, replaced by new cells. Some cells in hours, some can take longer, on average between every 11 to 18 months new cells arrive. If

this be the case, you might wonder; why are we getting older and falling apart? It is because our cells have a cellular memory.

The best way I know how to explain it is like this: each cell is assigned a specific job. For instance, a cell in the right little finger is only responsible for the right little finger. Beginning in the womb, the first cell has certain experiences that it then records as cell memory. Information on how to survive. Each cell, when it dies, passes along the information it has stored in its cellular memory to subsequent cells which come to replace it. The information from the previous cells; gets passed on from one cell to the next all the way throughout our life. Look at a person's finger as they age. Some people's history in their finger's maybe that of a broken, crooked, scared or discolored finger. This is their history!

There is a true story of a person who received an organ transplant, who after the transplant, that person suddenly started having cravings for a particular hamburger. He never had that hankering for them before. Come to find out, the organ donor had a habit and a great love of eating these particular hamburgers. This is an example of cell memory.

A teacher, who teaches a form of bodywork, told his class a story about Genghis Khan and his warriors. He said the reason they were so successful at conquering a great portion of the world is that they were fearless. After going to battle and being injured, they would do bodywork on each other. This would release the fear locked into those injured parts. The body cell memories of fear and survival, was in a sense, "ERASED" and their bodies would be ready to do battle the next day. I do not know if this story is true or not, but it does illustrates my point.

I like to think about cellular memory as a two year old and the brain as the parent. The two year old wants its way with all its bad habits. Then grows up, perhaps doing drugs or working too hard, not exercising, and eating unhealthy or has no joy in its life. The two year old (the cell) is trying hard to survive, but the parent (the brain) has not done well up to this point. Don't give up! It's not too late….For new cells are arriving soon. The brain, with some work and retraining can become a good parent once again. The tools in this book are great ways for the brain to regain control and retrain the cellular memory.

DON'T GIVE UP! IT IS NEVER TOO LATE, NEW CELLS ARE ARRIVING SOON.

⇒⋙ • ⋘⇐

Technique
SIMPLE BRAIN HEALTH

One of the simplest ways to protect your brain is by walking briskly daily for 20 minutes. A new British study suggests that by this 20 minute brisk walk cuts the risk of dementia and Alzheimer's disease in half. After age of 50, your brain memory centers begin getting 1% smaller each year, unless you start exercise regularly. The study shows that if you exercise your brain, memory center will grow 2% bigger every year, and helps keep its long and short term memory intact. Exercise stimulates the release of nerve growth factors, a chemical that is essential for the growth of healthy new brain cells.

Another very good way to keep the brain healthy is SLEEP. Getting seven to eight hours of restful sleep nightly halts brain aging and memory loss in as little as one month. Sleep is when the brain produces melatonin, a hormone that helps heal a damaged brain cell. Even if you don't make a single change, in your diet, exercise or lifestyle style habits, just aiming for seven hours of uninterrupted nightly sleep, can double your output of this healing hormone, melatonin. Your brain signals to the body to produce melatonin in the darkness, for best results keep your bedroom dark.

⇒⋙ • ⋘⇐

Technique
Releasing

Grief and unwanted aspects of our life that we are still carrying!

- Dear stomach, Linda can feel you growling so she knows it's time to get good food.

- Dear stomach, Linda knows you want a donut or something else sweet.
- Dear stomach, Linda knows what foods will be good for you.
- Dear stomach, food is on the way.
- Dear stomach, tell the rest of the body that good food is coming, as soon as Linda can fix it.
- Dear stomach, Linda will feed you as soon as Linda finds a quiet safe place to eat.
- Dear Linda, it is OK to feel abandon when you are hungry and need to be feed.
- Dear Linda, I know you can make wise choices with the food you are fixing.
- Dear Mom, why didn't you feed Linda when she got hungry?
- Dear Mom, when you were pregnant, what reason did you have for not eating better, so that Linda could be nourished better?
- Dear Mom, why were you not a responsible mother when you were pregnant with Linda?

Linda has eating problems. Linda was born with rickets and was never a fat baby or fat as a child. However, in her 40's, 50's and 60's, she was very overweight. Linda's mother never liked to eat and was extremely thin. Did they both have an eating disorder? Of course they did.

This process works for any obstacle you want to remove from your life, or an area you want to heal. Write at least two pages a day on any one subject, or several subjects. When you do so, don't write any answers to your DEARS. Do not write "ME" or "I." You don't want to own the unwanted stuff! You want to be able to release your grief. In writing your Dears, you want to release the grief and unwanted feelings and memories. This process is used to get them out of your subconscious. Whatever is not working for us, we need to remove it. Doing so we make room for what we do want. If you are filled up with unwanted issues or grief, there is no room for joy or the good stuff that life can bring you. You will be amazed by what you find out while writing the Dears.

I learned this process several years ago from a nurse in a grief support group. I have shared it with many people, including psychologists and family counselors. Again, don't answer any of the questions you are writing about. Just keep writing the Dears and all of the questions will be revealed, on their own, in due time. Use the name of another person, as I did in Dear Mom or an object, as I, did Dear stomach, along with your name. Do not use, "I" or "me" anywhere in your Dears.

I was having trouble paying my doctor and hospital bill over several months time. So I got out my pen and notebook, and starting writing. I just couldn't get enough money together. Even trying to make out the checks was so emotional for me. Here is a part of what I wrote.

- Dear Linda, why can't you save enough money to pay your doctor Bill?
- Dear Linda, why do you get so upset when you make out the check to make a payment on your doctor Bill?
- Dear Linda, what do you need to do to pay off your hospital Bill?
- Dear Hospital, why is the Bill so high?

After writing a full page, I looked over my writing and realized that all of the words "Bills" were written with a capital "B" instead of a small "b." My ex-husband's name was Bill! As soon as I recognized that, I knew I was not paying my doctor or hospital bills, I was still unconsciously paying my ex-husband alimony when I was making out the checks. As I told some friends my story, they recommended that I call the bills, "invoices" instead. The very next month both the doctor and hospital invoices were paid in full. Now, whenever I put a capital "B" in a word in the middle of a sentence, I stop myself and change it to a small "b." Depending on what I am writing about in that sentence, sometimes it is hard for me to write a small "b." My hand might cramp up, or I may get nervous, but now I am aware that I need to take notice of what is going on in my thoughts. I can heal, if I am aware.

Getting our grief under control is so important. Research has found that by the time we are 30 years old, if we haven't worked on letting go of things, we have more than enough grief to have a miserable, unhealthy life in our future. This process of writing the Dears is an easy way to release whatever we choose. It is clear, clean and easy. You may get answers while writing, but don't answer any of your questions, just write the questions. After a page of writing, you may look at the page and there the answer is, in the questions. Maybe later on, you may get the answers when you hear a song, hear a story, smell something – who knows! By doing the writings you will release whatever you no longer need and make room for something better. You will keep what you do need and your life will become much more beautiful. Life's journey is a beautiful thing. Give yourself a chance to fully live your journey!

⇛ • ⇚

Technique
Get up every half hour. Don't sit too long!

Stretch your body while you are watching TV, reading, or when you are sitting for long periods of time. When you are hurting, before taking a pill, get up and stretch. I mean, really stretch every muscle in your body. Make your stretches long and slow. Whatever you do on one side of your body, do on the other side of your body in the same way, even if only one side of your body is hurting. By doing both sides, it will balance your body and at the same time balance your brain.

⇛ • ⇚

Technique
Stretch before getting out of bed in the morning!

Lie on your back, keeping your shoulders flat on the bed, now, take your right leg and stretch it over the left leg, your goal is to go over and put the knee on the bed. Don't forget to keep your shoulder flat on the bed while stretching your right leg. Still keeping your shoulders flat on the bed, now, take your left leg and stretch it over the right leg, your goal is to go over and put the knee on the bed. Don't forget to keep your shoulder flat on the bed while stretching your left leg. Do not hold your leg in the stretched position, just touch the bed then do the other leg. Go back and forth three or four times.

At first, you may not be able to go all the way over and touch your knee to the bed. It could take several weeks or months to accomplish this goal. This exercise will get the body working in a healthy way, including the brain, our master computer for the body. This stretching will help with lower back, hip and knee pain. Then take each arm and stretch above your head several times. There have been several studies on heart attacks, and the results show that 70% of all heart attacks happen before 10 am in the morning. The results showed that the body becomes stagnant through the night. Stretching gently, jump starts the body and brain before getting out of bed.

Stretching benefits your health at anytime by:
1. Improves flexibility and brings health to the muscles, tendons and ligaments.
2. Stimulates blood circulation and moves the lymph's system, which helps to eliminates metabolic waste.
3. Breaks down friction and stickiness in the fascia sheathing.
4. Separates fibrosis and breaks down adhesions that may result from traumas and inflammation.
5. Reduces muscle spasms.
6. Reduces the risk of muscle strains and tears.

Please take note, "More is not better." Just do the stretches a few at a time. Take it slow. Doing stretches for just a few minutes will give you a much happier, stress free body.

⇉ • ⇇

Technique
Keep Your Brain Healthy!
Soft Cold Water Bottle (do not freeze)

One of the easiest ways to give the nerves a chance to communicate, to the correct part of your brain, is to place a room- temperature soft plastic water bottle behind your neck, resting the bottle under your neck at the base of your skull. This eases inflammation in the neck, supports the vertebrae and gives the muscles and tendons a chance to relax. It also reduces any swelling, helps the lymph glands to drain and in turn allows the nerves to signal to the correct part of the brain.

You do this by laying flat on the floor or bed with the cold water bottle behind your neck, for no more than 15 to 20 minutes at a time. You can use the cold water bottle several times a day but no more than 15 to 20 minutes at a time. When you are finished, stand up slowly and do some simple easy stretches.

As you look over the spine chart, you will see that each vertebra is responsible for protecting different nerves for different parts of the body. The nerves from each vertebra need to communicate to the correct part of the brain. If the correct message gets to the correct part of the brain, the brain will communicate back to the body telling it to heal itself. If we help our body to communicate, through the nerves, to the brain, then the brain will do its work. We have all heard that the body can heal itself, which is partly true. The human body constantly faces attack, from foreign invaders, that cause infection and disease. If the brain gets the proper communication, it will not send its whole Army Infantry to do a job, if the body only needs a Navy Seal to accomplish a particular defensive action. However, if we have had so many traumas in an area of our body that the brain says "that's enough" then it won't respond, and shuts off the sensation of pain. Another scenario is the possibility that nerve response did not get to the correct part of the brain to do any good. However, if our brain is healthy enough to act as a parent and not let that two year old cellular memory keep acting up and trying to get their way, our brain will help our body heal. We need to keep our brain healthy.

The top two bones of the spine are C1 (atlas) and C2 (axis) they are what support the head and are what the head balances on. The brainstem opening, at the base of the skull, is called the (foramen magnum). Another job of C1 and C2 is to protect the delicate brainstem without causing any interference to the nerves.

The brainstem houses all of the organ control centers. Every nerve we have either comes through here or originates from here.

AFFECT THIS AREA AND YOU CAN AFFECT EVERY AREA OF YOUR BODY FOR GOOD OR FOR BAD, IN SICKNESS OR IN HEALTH. It is your choice.

If you have TMJ or suffer a whiplash, you can place a cold gel pack on your tailbone and up the spine a ways, at the same time you are using the cold water bottle behind your neck. Again, gently stretch afterwards and you can do this several times a day for pain. One of the best times to use it, is a half hour before bedtime.

Note, when you get a whiplash, think of Indiana Jones with his whip. His hand is your tailbone and the tip of the whip is your neck. Depending on how hard he uses his hand (tailbone), the harder the tip of the whip snaps (your neck). If you have headaches, eye, ear, throat and sinus problems, you can get some relief using a cold water bottle behind the neck. By using this cold water bottle technique for 15 to 20 minutes, at least once a day, you will give yourself a great gift of relaxation and some much needed quiet time.

When I am driving for a half hour or longer, I put one bottle behind my neck between the seat and headrest, so it will not fall, if I move my head, and another one in front of my air conditioning vent, which I exchange out when the other one gets warm. This way, my TMJ will not give me any problems and I arrive at my destination without a headache.

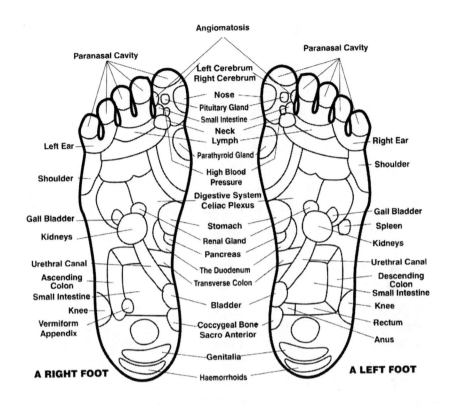

Angiomatosis

Paranasal Cavity

Paranasal Cavity

Left Cerebrum
Right Cerebrum

Nose
Pituitary Gland
Small Intestine
Neck
Lymph
Parathyroid Gland

High Blood
Pressure

Digestive System
Celiac Plexus

Stomach
Renal Gland
Pancreas

The Duodenum
Transverse Colon

Bladder

Coccygeal Bone
Sacro Anterior

Genitalia

Haemorrhoids

Left Ear

Shoulder

Gall Bladder
Kidneys

Urethral Canal
Ascending
Colon
Small Intestine
Knee
Vermiform
Appendix

A RIGHT FOOT

Right Ear

Shoulder

Gall Bladder
Spleen
Kidneys

Urethral Canal
Descending
Colon
Small Intestine
Knee
Rectum
Anus

A LEFT FOOT

➤➤ • ⋘

Technique
Golf Ball
(a form of reflexology you can do yourself)

Put a golf ball on the floor and roll it back and forth underneath your foot. Also, move your ankle and roll the ball to the right and left each way four or five times, roll the ball under your toes and on your heal, if you can. If there are some places on the foot that are tender or sensitive, do not dig or push hard on the area. Important, "do not use" the golf ball more than one or two minutes at a time on each foot. You can do this several times a day but only one to two minutes at a time.

If you were ever told to use another kind of ball, it may be for other purposes. I have heard that a tennis ball can be used or some fancy, expensive ball can be used. Try the golf ball and study a reflexology chart to figure out what is going on with your feet as well as your body.

➤➤ • ⋘

Technique
Salt Bath or Salt Shower!

A salt bath is preferred, but if you do not have a bathtub you can get some relief by taking a salt shower. You do not need any fancy salt just plain table salt will do. The purpose of a salt bath or shower is to release toxins from the body, not add to them. In a bath use about half of a regular size container of salt in the water. Keep the parts of the body wet that are not submerged and add salt on those areas. Stay in the bathtub for about 15 to 20 minutes if possible and relax. If you do not have a bathtub, use the shower. Get your whole body wet, including your hair, put a couple of tablespoons of salt on your wet hair where your baby soft spot was and leave it there. Wash your body as usual, then wash your hair as usual. Turn off the water and start at hairline with salt in your hand and rub the salt over your skin. Keep adding salt to your hand as needed. Go all the way down your body rubbing the salt both on the front and back of your body. When you are finished, rub your feet in the salt at the bottom of shower then rinse your body. This will exfoliate your skin, open pores, and rid your body of pollutants that are lying on the skin surface, plus cleanse the unwanted energy that you may have picked up during the day. You will feel very refreshed and relaxed.

➤➤ • ⋘

Technique
Joy Bank

Every day deposit joy in your Joy Bank. The joy bank is like a savings account. A savings account is for the unexpected financial needs in life. Things we did not plan on or expected would happen but did. Like money, JOY can be deposited into our account so when unexpected negative things happen to us, we have a reserve to get us through. My Joy Bank looks like an old eighteen hundred vault safe in an old bank that is standing strong. It is black, painted with rich gold lettering. The bank/vault is clean and fresh inside and outside, with many shelves on the inside. As I walk into the safe vault, I notice some of the shelves are filled with joy. However, there are many shelves without joy on them, having room for more joy to be added. I view this vault often. It is a reminder to look for and recognize my joy.

Sometimes I may not have noticed the joy that has come my way. I may have to go out and look for it. I deposit that joy, keeping my Joy Bank as full as I can. This way I have my joy savings account to help keep me happy and moving forward. Also, I add joy's that are just everyday life things, starting, with Nature. Nature is easy: birds singing, freshness after a good rain. Other favorites: a hot cup of coffee, or an unexpected call from someone. Whatever brings me joy; I put it into my Joy Bank. If something comes along that is really taking a lot of joy out of me (taking joy out of my bank), I must replenish it as soon as possible. By putting joy into my Joy Bank, my Joy Bank becomes an "artesian well" of joy. If circumstances weigh me down, if I am troubled or hurting, I go to the Joy Bank. If I am lonely or afraid, I go to my Joy Bank. It is my every flowing "artesian well" of joy. Sure I get sad, afraid, hurt, angry, lonely, mad and guilty. I feel all of these emotions. I do not dismiss these emotions or hide from them. I mean, I really feel them. I may feel them all day, or just an hour or whatever time I need to really feel them. Then off to my beautiful black vault with the bright gold lettering and look at what joy has been deposited there. I am human and just like the rest of you, I need to learn from these emotions, but I don't have to keep them hanging around.

→»» • «←

Technique
Find JOY in Your Life

Listen to a sad song; it gets you out of a funk, fast. Next time you feel a little down; try listening to a sad song such as, Susan Boyle's "I Dream a Dream" or Roy Orbison's "Crying" or Elton

John's "Sad Songs Say So Much." It may seem counterintuitive, but the beauty of sad songs draws you in so much that it shifts your focus to the lyrics and melody and away from whatever spurred your funk in the first place.

Scary movies like The Shining, Psycho and Silence of the Lambs get your pulse racing and heart beating. Then there is a sense of relief you feel when the scary parts are over. This triggers a surge of good feelings that make you happy long after the movie is over.

Research shows the following:

1. Sharing your story of a setback or something you are not happy about will help you overcome them much faster. If they are shared with friends and family to get support, it helps defuse the negative feeling quickly.
2. Next time something positive happens, such as: your grown son calls you first before anyone else about his good news, or you receive a compliment on your front yard garden from your neighbor. Do what happy people do, tell other people all about it. You can share in person, by phone, on Twitter or Facebook and any other social media. Sharing this news makes you feel twice as good as you would have if you had kept it to yourself. Why? Because it makes your good fortune more prominent in your own mind and you think about it more throughout the day.

Looking back can make for a brighter future. Do you think living in the past will make you sad? Forget it. The happiest people think about the past all the time and this leads them to a brighter future." By remembering your successes from the past, your achievements and the challenges you've overcome, this remembering actually enhances your belief that you are worthy of having good things in your life. Looking ahead lengthens your life. People, who expect to have positive experiences in the future, are not only happier, they live 7.5 years longer. Focus on the positive for what lies ahead, especially as you get older. Having fewer responsibilities and more time for hobbies inspires people to adopt healthy habits now.

Writing this poem has given me joy and, of course fishing, does too.

When I Go Fishing

The boat rocks calmly as I step in
Softly the engine moves the boat away from the dock.
The warmth of the slick worm wraps around my finger
as I put it on the hook.
Woosh goes the fish line,
glistening in the sun as the bobber lands in the water.
The fish line relaxes; I relax listening
to the outdoors and smelling nature in the air.
Then I see the bobber go under, the line gets tight
and the sound of the reel is a glorious sound.
As I reel the fish in,
out comes the net as I pull the fish closer to the boat.
Seeing the beauty of this stripped fish, I say
"Hi" as I look into the fish's eyes.
What a marvelous creature!
Gently I remove the hook from his mouth,
carefully not to damage his mouth in any way.
Then slowly I lean down and gently place the fish
back into the cool water.
Freedom.....as he swims away!

⇒⇒ • ⇐⇐

Technique
Write 10 Successful Things You Have Done in your Life

Write 10 things that you have done successfully. The list should include things that you have been successful doing at any age: as a child, as a parent, dating, in marriage, at work etc. Write successful things that really mean something to you. Things you really had to work hard at to accomplish a successful outcome. Keep the list handy at all times. If you need to figure out how to handle whatever is happening to you now, or something that is getting you down, you have a template. You can see how you handled some past thing and turned it into a success. Even if the current challenge may not be exactly like one of your successes on the list, the list can be an example of how to handle the challenge now. The brain maybe unable to create an instant response when first faced with a challenge or until a situation calms down. However, if you have the list handy, you can instantly start taking action to get a successful outcome. Use your past successes to move towards a healthy outcome.

➔≫ • ≪←

Technique
Protein
(Check with your health care professional)

Protein is used to construct, maintain and repair most tissue in our bodies: brain, bones, teeth, muscles, nerves, glands, heart, liver, skin, hair and everything in between. The lack of protein is mostly associated with muscle weakness, slow healing and brain chemistry imbalance. An excess of animal protein is associated with heart and kidney disease, cancers, including colon cancer. Use fish and plant base protein when possible. Next to water, protein makes up the greatest portion of body weight and builds nearly all aspects of the microscopic cellular machinery. It is essential to the growth of bones. Proteins themselves, can act as neurotransmitters or precursors to neurotransmitters enabling all our cells to receive and transmit messages. The absence of the amino acid, tryptophan, leads to a deficiency in serotonin. The body will create serotonin from tryptophan. Serotonin is essential for generating feelings of well-being a stress defense shield that helps cope with hardships, depression, chronic stomach problems and neurological disorders.

➔≫ • ≪←

Technique
Insomnia

When you can't sleep or can't get back to sleep late at night, take a hand towel and fold it length wise into thirds. Pull it tight, over the eyes, and tuck it at the back and base of the skull. This does several things. It keeps all light out of the eyes, muffles sounds and puts pressure on the nerves as they go to the brain to settle them down. Professor Temple Grandin learned, as a young girl to quiet her body down by applying pressure. She famously used this principal as an adult to calm down cattle. Try it, it may give you calmness, as you try to go back to sleep. If you wake up in the middle of the night, thinking about something, keep a notepad by your bed and jot down a few words. Don't turn on the light. The few words will remind you in the morning. Write it down first and then put the towel over your eyes.

⇒⇒ • ⇐⇐

Technique
Urinary Problems

Many people get up several times during the night and are unable to get a good REM sleep. Studies have shown that people over 50 do not get thirsty until later in the day. Our body tissue is like a sponge. If a sponge is dry and you try and wipe some liquid up, the sponge will not absorb the liquid. However, if the sponge is wet, it will absorb the liquid and then you can squeeze it out (eliminate) and then it will absorb some more. Your cells need to stay hydrated, especially the brain. Hydration is important to keep the brain healthy and active. So if you are over 50 years old, you really need to start drinking water in the morning. Remember coffee and caffeine drinks dehydrate the body and the brain, so if you are trying to get hydrated, do not drink too much caffeine.

It is also important to check and see if you have a blocked airway, or snore when sleeping. If you can't catch your breath during sleep, the brain can't rest and will not let the body go into REM sleep. The body thinks it has to function as if you were awake. If the brain tells the body to function as if it is awake and you drink most of your liquids after 3pm your kidneys and bladder think they have to function all through the night, keeping you up. Please get a sleep study done to see if you need a C-pap to help you get good sound sleep at night. I prefer the test that is done in your own home, instead going to a sleep center. Surprisingly, a C-pap has proven to help with Urinary Problems. Remember that the brain needs enough sleep to stay healthy and so does the body. You need time to rest!

REM sleep is a rapid, periodic jerky movement of the eyes during certain stages of the sleep cycle, when dreaming takes place.

Do you remember how to do your Kegel exercises, this too, could help. This exercise is recommended for men also. Can't remember the Kegel exercise? Look it up on the internet.

⇒⇒ • ⇐⇐

Technique
Drinking Enough Water!

How do you know if you are drinking enough water and getting that water into your body's cells?

Consult with your health care professional to see if you are healthy enough, before doing anything about hydration on your own. Your medication or health condition may warrant a different approach.

Signs of dehydration:
1. Are you tired? Water can boost your energy level.
2. Gaining weight? Water can help you control your appetite and keep calorie intake down.
3. Joint pain? Water lubricates your joints and can alleviate pain.
4. Your immune system weak? Water propels hydration and can help prevent coughs, colds and flu.
5. Your skin looks or feels bad? Water keeps your skin from looking and feeling dry and skin dehydration causes wrinkles.
6. Dry hard stools? Water can soften your body tissue and soften stools to make elimination easier and complete.

Not all liquid can be considered beneficial as water, caffeinated drinks, such as sodas, coffee and some teas are dehydrating. So how can you know if you are getting enough water? This rule applies to most- take your weight, divide it in half and that is how many ounces of water you need to drink each day to stay hydrated. If you have been dehydrated based on the above signs, it is important not to drink water too fast. Your body cells are like a sponge and a dry sponge will not take in liquid. However, if it is moist, it will drink in that liquid. So to get your cells to drink, drink 1oz. of water every 15 minutes and start early in the day to get most of your water intake by 3pm. Do this for two weeks to get the cells hydrated. If you have heart or kidney trouble, or your healthcare professional advises you to watch your liquid intake, do not drink this much water. Please check with your healthcare professional on the amount and the ways they advise you to take in liquid. As we age, people over 50 years old drink most of their liquid late in the day. This can cause many health issues, including having to get up in the middle of the night to urinate often. By drinking your liquids, starting in the morning soon after waking, you will keep the whole body functional and it will be easier to stay balanced. You can get hydration strips at a health food store if you have any concerns. These strips are different than the pH strips.

⇻ • ⇺

Technique
Checking Your pH Level

Your pH level needs to be 7.0. When it is, you will have less health issues. Below 6.4 is too acidic and above 7.2 is too alkaline. When you wake up in the morning and before you eat or drink any liquids, spit into a spoon, then put in the pH stick. If you are using your urine, check it the first time you urinate in the morning. Check it every day for a month, until you know how to keep it around 7.0 easily. Watch what you drink and eat, but also watch what is in the cleaning solutions, toxins you touch and what you breathe in. This monitoring will determine any important diet or lifestyle changes you may need to take. After following your pH levels for a month, then check it every week to stay healthy. You can get the strips at most drug and health food stores.

⇒⇒ • ⇐⇐

Technique
Alcohol spray

Spray rubbing alcohol all around you whenever you feel tired, drained by others, need to be uplifted or you feel that you need a bath but can't get one right away. This will change the energy around you and you will feel lighter, refreshed and at peace. Close your eyes and just spray the air around you about 12 inches away from your body. You can also use the spray on your hands and spray things others have touched. If you want to stay clean and do not want to pick up something from others, try using the alcohol spray. I have seen people use vodka with lavender oil as a substitute since some people are allergic to rubbing alcohol. I have my spray with me at all time, so I do not use vodka. If I am really busy and a part of my body is hurting, I will spray the alcohol right where it hurts and sometimes that will release the pain.

⇒⇒ • ⇐⇐

Technique
"Colors and Numbers" Book
by Louise L. Hay

Balance the body by using your own numbers; your birthday, plus current year and month. It is exciting to see people who use this idea for several months or years, to see how their lives have changed. This is a great way to stay healthy and have your life work for you. It keeps your energy level up, keeps you calmer and keeps you in a healthy pattern flow in an easy simple way. You chart out the month with a color of the day. On your days color, you wear and read the message of the day. The colors rotate throughout the month, along with the message. It is easy to apply in your life and the rewards are exceptional.

Technique
"The 7 Principles of Fat Burning"
by Eric Berg, DC

The book is a complete guide to understand what your body is lacking and why your body is not functioning properly. It is an easy read and very helpful. It discusses the reasons for your current health condition. It will explain why some diets don't work for you but work for others. You will not feel like a failure after reading this book. Don't forget to take the simple test inside. I recommend this book, no matter what diet you want to use. This book will empower you. It will explain why you might need to prepare your body, so you can be successful in dieting and even more important, why you have not been successful in keeping the pounds off. Even though it is a diet book it is important to do the liver support drink first, before starting any diet. It is important to get the liver strong and healthy. The liver can rejuvenate itself if you allow it. If you take the time to understand what is written in this book, you can see why your body looks and acts like it does. It is not because of a lack of will power, it's because of your body's imbalance. The fear of gaining weight will be lifted, and the negative self-talk tapes you have been running in your mind will be lifted. Can't gain weight, you might want to read this book..

➺➺ • ⋘

Technique
"Chinese and Western Astrology" Book
by Suzanne White

I really like this author's style of writing, because it is easy and simple to understand both your Chinese Astrology animal sign and your Western Astrology sign, which are both great astrological systems that many people use. She explains that there are not just twelve Chinese Astrology signs but 144 signs, and then combines them with the twelve Western Astrology signs. It is a serious tool for awareness and understanding of oneself, providing a great way to see our strengths and weaknesses, and to better understand our life and purpose. This book is not intended to help you live your day to day life, like your own personal chart would, but makes us aware why we do the things we do and why we like the things we like. We all have a monkey mind at times, but those born under the Chinese Astrology sign of the Monkey, are far more likely to hear that monkey mind.

I am a Sagittarius and a Rooster. The Rooster is the first to wake up. Then the Rooster's duty is to wake up the barnyard, getting all the animals, the farmer, his family going at the same time each day come rain or shine. All my life I have been with other Roosters growing up, in school and beyond into adulthood. How many Roosters in a barnyard? "ONE" If there is more than one in the barnyard you have a cock fight. I have had many years of practice solving conflicts, defusing fights and taking charge.

A Sagittarian is half human and half horse. So that makes me someone who likes adventure and likes to travel. I can go beyond human thinking and successfully think outside the box. This energy shows up in my creativity. All through my life I have been a teacher and a student at the same time. I am a good networker. I can find value in everyone and I connect people together. People and Nature are more important to me than material things, but I do like beauty and balance around me. I can entertain as a good hostess, offering fun and laughter with everything I do. Work is serious to me, but I put fun into my work. I have had many firsts in my life, both personally and career wise.

⇛ • ⇚

Technique
"Take Five: The Five Elements Guide of Health
and Harmony" Book by Pamela Ferguson

This book is a guide on health by living in harmony with the five elements. It shows us how to use the links between the seasonal cycles and our body, moods, foods and colors. It gives us insight and ways to harmonize our meridians to counter the effects of toxins and pollutants. This is a workbook style of writing with color-coded step by step processes that are easy to follow. Good health is a free flowing of energy through a balanced lifestyle of nutrition, exercise, meditation, consciousness and discipline. A good life bundles all these aspects.

➤➤ • ◄◄

Technique
Meditation

The benefits of meditation range from the simple and obvious, to greater physical relaxation, and the subtle, less known inner stillness. All meditation supports the body and brain, increases energy and improves health. It is a mental exercise that helps you achieve deep relaxation of the mind and body through carefully controlled breathing. By breathing deeper and deeper, the chatter of your monkey mind subsides, which leads to a deep healing state.

Meditation helps you circumvent the fight or flight response, which is a set of involuntary bodily reactions that includes: increased adrenalin production, faster heart rate and higher blood pressure. This natural response originates in the oldest part of the brain developed by our prehistoric ancestors. That is a result in our unconscious, mindless survival instincts to kick in as either fight – meeting the threat of an aggressor with similar aggression – or to flight – running away from our aggressor.

Research has uncovered that stress and negative thoughts like fear, anxiety and anger, produces the same physiological, neurological and endocrinological changes in the body, as does the fight or flight response. The fight or flight response is hardwired in the brain to act on a threatening situation and to be used only for short periods, once in a while. When this becomes the normal response to everyday life, it leads to serious health issues. Studies have shown that meditation does just the opposite of fight or flight to the body, thereby promoting good health. Meditation sharpens one's mental faculties, improves attention span and enhances the ability to stay focused for longer periods of time.

Throughout the day, you can do a 5 to 15 minute meditation to keep your mind, body and emotions balanced. Close your eyes and go within. Taking a few cleansing breaths, it allows your sense of burden to melt away. Focus on the gentle rise and fall of your chest and abdomen as you inhale and exhale. As you go deeper, experience your oneness with life. Every cell of your body is filled with life force. Every aspect of who you are is an expression of creation. Let yourself feel at peace. Then new insights and ideas will fill you with infinite options and ideas.

This is how I meditate: I sit quietly and begin by focusing on my breath. I breathe in and think of being at peace. I breathe out and I let go of stress. I notice my breath flowing into each part of: my body, my head, my shoulders and my chest. I breathe out through my arms, down my torso, and all the way out the bottoms of my feet. My heart, mind and body can feel the energy flowing in me with ease. After a few minutes, I bring my attention back to where I am sitting. I return to my activities with more clarity.

When I was pregnant, I worked on my feet for eight hours and my whole body got tired. So on my breaks and at lunch, I would meditate to get much needed rest. I still had to drive an hour in traffic to get home and cook and clean. I enjoyed my meditation sessions, since it was just me and my baby meditating together.

Even if you don't feel you can learn to meditate, you can still boost your longevity by closing your eyes and thinking positive thoughts about others. Reap the benefits by finding a comfortable place and sit quietly for 10 minutes; ideally in the morning when your mind is the clearest. Focus on your loved ones. Think about the warmth you feel for that person and focus on the happy memories you had with the person. In addition to feeling calmer afterwards, you will be more optimistic about the future. Brain scans show that happy memories spark activity in the emotional region of the brain.

⇛ • ⇚

Technique
Acupressure Magic

Doing it yourself
Get hunger cravings?
If you are hungry and know you are about to face temptation,

start by taking a deep breath, draw your breath in slowly, as if your breath is going in the top of your head and then pushing your breath down your spine. Do this several times. Next, find the spot behind where your earlobe meets the skin and bone and gently rub in a circular motion, going first to the left three to four times and then to the right for about 30 seconds. Why does this work? This type of acupressure significantly improves your body's level of leptin, a hormone key to weight loss control. This technique not only improves leptin but also reduces hunger. Because leptin plays a role in blood sugar control, it can also decrease sugar cravings.

⇛ • ⇚

Technique
Out of Control Eating When You are Hungry or Stressed

Trigger the gallbladder to reduce and dissolve more fat. Before you start eating a meal, take a few deep breaths. Then begin using your fingertips and rub the muscles softly, like you would pet cat, in a circular motion along your jaw line. Start under your ear, down your chin and down your neck to your collarbone for 90 seconds. It hits the points that trigger the gallbladder to produce bile that naturally dissolves fat. It also engages the brain pathways that help relax the stomach. Doing this helps to prevent weight gain and gives you another way to take control of your life.

⇛ • ⇚

Technique
Boost your Metabolism

Hydrate with water first, if your energy is low. Often, it is a sign that you need to turn calories into fuel a little faster. Squeeze the little bump just above the ear opening with light pressure for a hold of 8 seconds and then release for 10 seconds; repeat several times. Then do exactly the same with the other ear to keep your brain balanced. This meridian corresponds to your endocrine system: including your thyroid and adrenal glands. These glands are responsible for regulating metabolism and releasing weight loss hormones.

⇒» • «⇐

Technique
Sleep like a Baby

When you are ready to go to sleep, hold your hand palm side up and use the thumb of your other hand to massage the half of your wrist closest to your pinky finger. Apply pressure and massaging for 90 seconds, then switch to the other wrist and do the same. In addition to this, you can try using a dark sleep mask to block out any light and the pressure on your eyes is a soothing experience as well.

⇒» • «⇐

Technique
TMJ Jaw and Joint Pain!

Give yourself a little mini massage while you are sitting at a traffic signal. I find my jaw gets tense and tight while driving. Place the tip of the tongue to the roof of your month and place your fingers of both hands at your nose just under your cheek bones. Push in with your fingers and up with your tongue at the same time then release. Move your fingers about ¼ inch towards your ear and repeat pushing in and up at the same time. Repeat all the way to your jaw hinge. This can be done several times a day or when needed.

For joint pain: you can get an immediate response to pain and you may find instant relief. This is for pain anywhere in the body, if that pain just came on. Take your left hand thumb and index finger, put them on the right hand between the right thumb and index finger where the webbing soft fatty tissue is and squeeze hard for 30 seconds. Then repeat on the other hand. Repeat several times. Sometimes this works very well.

Technique
Massage Therapy

Generally speaking about 80% of adults' ages 30 to 60 in the United States have reported suffering from back pain. Back pain tends to be more common among older adults. Health care professionals divide conditions into two categories based on the duration of the pain; acute and chronic. Either way, massage can help. Pain can be relieved by massage, especially as we get older. Over the years, accumulated improper lifting, sudden trauma, repeating work and unhealthy lifestyles, add to back pain. Some of the conditions that show up as we age in our back are: tingling, weakness or numbness in our legs, and can radiate in the lower back, leg and buttocks and can include muscle spasms.

Also, some other condition but not limited to are; muscle tenderness, dull achy pain, stiffness and limited range of motion. Degenerative disc disease can strike as early as 30, but more often 50 and older. This happens when proteins leaking from the compressed disc can irritate the adjacent nerve root.

Massages can help our body maintain flexibility and encourage blood flow, especially as we age. A massage therapist goal is to help clients feel better and return to normal levels of activity. A 2001 study showed that people having regular massages, report a greater reduction in pain, less depression and less anxiety and improved sleep. They also, had higher dopamine and serotonin levels in their blood. Massage along with self care, exercise and education, give clients good results and report of a significant reduction in pain.

I always stress that the whole body needs to be massaged, to make sure that there are not other muscles that may be involve with the pain. For lower back pain, other muscle groups include the gluteus, hamstrings, quadriceps, and hip flexors. If these muscle groups are imbalanced, they may be creating an uneven pull or torque on the lower back and pelvis that contributes to the pain.

Massage and stretches can help relieve pain. Some lower

back pain is related to poor body mechanics or compensating movement and poor posture because of existing pain. A massage therapist can help the client develop new habits and re-educate the neuromuscular pathways. Neuromuscular retraining is brain work, so it takes new movement and new stretching to get nerves firing in new ways. Massage therapist may collaborate with physicians, chiropractors, rehabilitation specialists, and other professionals for positive health outcomes.

A bit of history about massage coming to the United States: Massage therapy started in colonial times, back in the 1700's. Those doing the massage were called "rubbers", treating orthopedic problems by rubbing and creating heat in the body. In the 1850's medical gymnastics, were used to promote health, prevent disease and treat injuries. Swedish "movement" massage was scientific and holistic and still remains today. In fact, Swedish massage is the most commonly requested type of massage at spas today.

The title of masseuse or masseur became common in the 1880's referring to those using manual therapies. By the early 1900's massage became the dominant term. Massage and hydrotherapy are the treatments provided by many spas today. Treatments, such as body wraps and scrubs started in the late 1800's. By the 1890's advocates felt that natural approaches promoted good health and served as alternatives to conventional medicine. Massage therapy was used widely throughout the 1930's, 40's and 50's. The facilities were called massage parlors. However, soon the name was associated with prostitution.

By 1960 the professionals referred to themselves as massage therapists and practitioners of massage therapy. The term therapy was defined generally as promoting good health by encompassing a whole range of applications. The whole massage therapy practice went through a transformation between 1970 and 2000. Now it encompasses the "wellness movement", "fitness boom", concern about unhealthy stress and the growth of alternative medicine. Everyone can benefit from massage. Massage connects the brain, body and mind, at the same time, to give a natural approach to healing.

Technique
No More Hospital Corner at the Foot of Your Bed

I work with many modalities to determine what is going on with the body. I am not just looking at your knee because you have had a knee problem and it is getting worse. I use a lot of modalities at once. Remember your multiplications and division back in 3rd or 4th grade? To find out if our division answer was correct we just multiplied. There it was; the right answers!

As you use this book, you to, will find some easy ways to discover what causes your knees to ache and become swollen. It may be as easy as finding out that those hospital corners you have made on your bed all these years have been causing your knee problems today. Please stop using hospital corners for a month and see if it helps.

Place cold water bottles under each knee for 20 minutes. Relax as you are lying down with the cold water bottles. Take note on how you get up off the toilet or chair. Do you push on the top of your knee/leg? If so, stop. Think of your body as a fine gold chain necklace. If a fine gold chain necklace gets all tangled up, you don't go to the center of that necklace and start pulling at it. You go to the fringes, and work a little here, and a little there, until it is all untangled, you go easy and you don't rush to untangle it. That is pretty much what you may have to do when you have a health problem or pain in whatever area of the body. Go at it easy, and try a little here and a little there to get better.

⋙ • ⋘

Technique: *Our Body and the Seasons*

Our body has cycles just like the seasons of the year: Spring, Summer, Late Summer, Fall and Winter. Like the planting and caring of a crop, we too, can use the crop example; to better understand how we can care for our physical and emotional life for ourselves and our loved ones.

Our moods, thoughts, feelings and impulses, obsessions,

cravings, avoidances, don't just happen by chance. They are expressed and give useful insight into human behavior, whether chronic or cycles of acute health problems. All of which, may be linked to seasons and climates.

⇶ • ⇇

Men's vs. Women's Health

We can better understand women's and men's health by looking at some myths. Depression is not just a "woman's problem." One out of eight men is depressed. Heart disease was considered a "man's condition" and women were excluded from major studies until recently, even though heart disease is the number killer of women. There is an obsession in the US with breast cancer fund raisers. Every kind of event from cocktail parties to marathons, and street protests rally for more research on breast cancer, that hits one in eight women. Do you hear them mention that breast cancer hits 1% of the men?

Prostate cancer hits one in five men in the US.

⇶ • ⇇

Yin and Yang

It is the movement of stillness and the stillness of movement. Yin is stillness and Yang is movement not as opposites, but complements to each other. Yin and Yang are with us everyday throughout our lives. Like, but not limited to, the sun and the moon, dark and bright, night and day, hot and cold. It is in our Ph level and as we exhale and inhale. In German, sun is feminine and moon is masculine. In Latin America, the sun is masculine and moon is feminine. Electricity depends on a positive and negative charge.

A battery must line up with the plus or minus charge to work for you. When your car battery needs a jump the red color cable cover is Yang and the black color cable cover is Yin. The front of the body is Yin and back of the body is Yang. The Chi (energy) runs on meridians. The Yin runs from our feet to our head and the Yang run from our head to our feet. Yin organs are dense like the lungs, heart and kidneys. The Yang organs transport and are hollow like the large and small intestines and the bladder.

⇛ • ⇚

Technique
Hot Flashes or Being Extremely Cold

You can visually meditate by using any of these exercises to get results. If you've got hot flashes and can't sleep, picture yourself in the blue water of the ocean or picture a blue cloth wrapped around you. If you are extremely cold and can't get warm, picture a fire burning or picture the color red cloth wrapped around you.

Put Play back into your life: You think you are too old to play like a child? Play can lighten your body, lighten you mood, and lighten your life in general. If you feel silly or afraid to try; go do the following where no one can see you or don't know you.

Get a water gun and shoot the flowers and trees. Find a site and go for it. Have a dog? Shoot towards his mouth, I guarantee he will open his mouth to try and catch the water. Water balloons work the same, except not with the dog. Go where they rent bikes and rent one by the hour or half hour. After renting a bike for a few times you may have the courage to ask a friend to come along with you. Even people using a cane can rent a three wheel bike.

Not many playground areas have swings anymore, but go looking, you may find one. Start slow when swinging, and if there are other people around, don't worry. They don't know you and you will never see them again. Go out into nature or to a park, whip out your coloring book and color markers. Color markers have bold color that stimulates the brain.

Once a month have a The Good Old Days luncheon. Dress up, play music, tell stories, be creative. Have fun and laugh a lot!

Chapter 18

11 Short Stories

The American aviatrix, Elinor Smith, once said, "It has come to my attention that people of accomplishment rarely sit back and let things happen to them. They went out and happened to things!"

M any of my clients and students have used the techniques in this book, here 11 more success stories!

Ms. D. writes: six years ago, I had a melanoma removed from my lower leg. During my semi-annual check-ups, I was always very careful about keeping an eye out for any changes in my skin. This last summer I was looking forward to my visit to Alaska when I noticed a tiny white lump right by my old melanoma scar. I thought, "I should get this checked before my trip, so I won't be worrying about it. I called the dermatology office and explained my situation. The receptionist dismissed me, saying, "I'm Sorry, we have no openings for two weeks." I was adamant that it be looked at. "Look," I said. "It is very important because of the previous melanoma, that I get this looked at now. It will just take a few minutes.""No", she replied. "We would still have to schedule an appointment." By this time I was getting angry and I said," Well, I'll just come down there and sit until he sees me!" "He still wouldn't see you without an appointment" she commented. That's when I hung up on her, which I have never done before.

The next morning, the office called me and said they had scheduled an appointment for me that day. I think she might have been talking about that "rude" woman, and the Doctor or nurse heard her and had her schedule me.

When I asked my doctor what he thought it was he said, "I have no idea, but we'll take it out and biopsy it. Four days later the biopsy came back. It was melanoma. The PET scan and the MRI of my whole body came back clear and so I will have surgery on it and monitor it as we did the first time.

I feel good that I was pro-active about this and I encourage everyone to take charge of their own health. If you don't, someone else will. You know your own body better than anyone.

Ms. D. wrote the following poem:

"The return"
Hello
I'm back
Where were you
All this time
Gone so long
Six years
I had forgotten about you
Not really
You were always
In the back
Of my mind
And now you have the nerve
To enter
My life
Again
And turn it topsy turvy around
Such a tiny white lump
Over an old scar
Who'da thought
The cancer has returned
Here we go again

Ms. M, Is now a retired 3rd grade teacher. She is a happy, active 70 year old. I have known Ms. M. for about 9 years. She has used many of the techniques that I have recommended. She uses the golf ball to keep her body in good working order. She uses her silk cloth to help keep her chronic pain under control. Ms. M. uses a cold water bottle behind her neck and behind her knees to reduce inflammation which keeps her lymph systems moving. Like most people, when she is feeling better, she forgets to use her cold water bottles but when the pain comes back she again starts using the cold water bottles. We are all human. We forget, or get lazy doing something good for us and then abandon it. Most importantly, Ms. M remembers to go back to what works for her. When she was a teacher, one of the most important things she used was Super Brain Yoga in her classroom. Ms. M. did her research and found it was simple and easy for many of the kids she had that year, who had learning problems. That was the year that a magazine came out with an article on Super Brain Yoga. One of her brightest students took Super Brain Yoga out to the playground and before long, students in the whole school were doing Super Brain Yoga before school started. Ms. M. found that some of her students, when they were having problems doing work in class, would stand up and do Super Brain Yoga and then resume doing their work without difficulty. It put a smile on her face seeing her students excel that way. Many years later she called and asked for a refresher on Super Brain Yoga so she could pass it on to her grandson who was having difficulty in school. I have seen many people of all ages do much better when using Super Brain Yoga.

Ms. G. An active married 60 year old woman drives a school bus for a living. She gets up early each morning before the sun comes up. She keeps a pretty good routine during the week and is very active on the weekends with family and friends. She took a class on colors and numbers from me, and has been using them for two years now. Oh, has her life changed! She starts on Sunday night placing tops and blouses in the colors she needs for the week and puts them in order. She usually wears jeans while working but her tops changes color. Monday top might be red, Tuesday orange, Wednesday yellow, Thursday green and Friday blue. On the weekends she has many options of clothing to wear but still uses her colors of the day. At first, she just used the color by wearing it as a blouse. Now she may wear a whole outfit in the color of the day and add other things to look at in those colors. She now uses what she calls a "cheat sheet" that lists the number, the color, and the key word and affirmations of the day. She uses her cheat sheet as a reference and continues to explore how she can use the colors and numbers in her everyday life. She knows some people even eat the colors of the day and she is now exploring that as well.

She remembered one Sunday, when she was volunteering at church, which she has done for many years. This Sunday just didn't seem right. Everything was a little off, even people she saw noticed. There just seemed to be more problems than normal. It continued throughout the day as she continued her activities. She realized that evening, that she was wearing the wrong color and focusing on the wrong number of the day. That day made her realize how much the color and number system really works for her.

Ms. G. says "I have found that this small habit of using colors and numbers and by developing them into my life has made a big difference. How smoothly my life seems to run and I am grateful." This color and number practice has led her to listen to her body. Now she takes time to do water aerobics and tei chi every other day and still gets in her walking. Most days her back and knees are pain free.

Ms. P. She met me about 10 years ago through her horse trainer. At 82 she was still riding horses and saddling them herself. She is about 5 feet tall and about 100 pounds. Ms. P. is a small lady for such a big horse. Her horse of 22 years recently died, just after her husband died. She has had many losses in the past few years, Sorry Ms. P. She eats very healthy foods, stays active on her mini farm; works in her garden and with her animals each and every day. She has many long time friends, stays active in church and Bible Study.

A little over a year ago she went on a two week pilgrimage to Israel with many of her church friends. She was moved by that experience. Oh yes, Ms. P. has fibromyalgia and has had it for most of her adult life. She uses a cold water bottle behind her neck. By riding her horse and walking all around her property, she has kept her lymph's moving. She does Super Brain Yoga first thing in the morning and during the day when she has pain. She is a really good mentor to her daughters and especially to her granddaughters. Ms P. has taught and shows her granddaughters how important massage is for good health, along with good diet, exercise, and a balanced life full of God, love and adventure. One of her granddaughters has become a massage therapist. I still work on her several times a year, when she needs a tune up. This woman has been an extremely good mentor to me and for many younger women.

Ms. S. Her attorney introduced her to me more than 15 years ago. She is a beautiful single mom with two children, in her late 40s. She is a stylish dresser and has her nails and hair done on a regular basis. She works in a very powerful position and has a very active social life. Ms. S. was born with scoliosis, but never had any medical care for it as a child. She has spinal stenosis and degenerative disease in her spine and both knees.

She does a self massage with a medical machine at least once a day. Takes salt baths and showers several times a week. She uses the alcohol spray as needed. She has changed her diet, changed her shoes, she uses the cold water bottle behind her neck when driving home from work. She alternates cold to hot to cold to hot to cold therapy on her feet when needed, and gets massages and body work regularly. She stretches before going to bed and before getting out of bed in the morning.

Ms. S. has had to listen to her body to prevent injuries, and she keeps her pain under control. She tries to live a balanced life, but sometimes does not get the rest she needs. She is a very courageous woman when it comes to being proactive for herself and the health of her two children. There isn't anywhere in her body she does not have pain because of her spine. She has been dealing with pain all her life and still is able to maintain a pretty normal life.

Mr. M. He was in his mid 50s when I first saw him. A man well over six feet tall, built like a football player. Every morning, for years, he and his wife go running to keep in shape and train to compete in races they do together several times a year. These runs and getting older have been hard on his knees. His legs would cramp up often and the pain gave him grief. Mr. M. went to his primary doctor, who sent him to an orthopedic doctor, who sent him to a physical therapist, also went to a chiropractor every once in awhile.

When I saw him I took one look at the calves of his legs. Then I asked him "What do your doctors say about the condition of your muscles in your legs?" He said "None of them said anything about the muscles, why?" I thought for awhile and then said "Your legs look like an old wash board. The scaring in your legs looks like it has been there for a long time. It kind of looks like when you were a young boy you might have put a towel around your neck and jumped off the fence or a roof trying to be Superman." He laughed and said "I know just what happened. When I was a small boy my grandmother made me a Superman cape so I could be Superman. I didn't jump off of fences. I would jump out of the loft of our barn and sometimes missed the hay!"

He did not want to stop running with his wife, although I suggested not running any more. He also, didn't want to stop competing in races. I knew I would not see him for at least three months, so I gave him something he could to do for himself in the meantime. I would check on him when I got back.

Three months went by and I was back to see him. I looked at his legs and asked, Mr. M. what on earth have you been doing? He asked "NOW WHAT's WRONG!" Nothing, your legs look so much better. What have you been doing? "Well, you told me to cool off my leg muscles by taking a cool shower after running. That did not seem to work for us. When my wife and I get through running, she goes in and takes her shower and I go into our pool up to my waist and cool my leg muscles down. I feel better and at our last race competition, we won a metal." I only saw him two more times. He has gotten older, but he still runs with his wife and wins metals.

Ms. G. We were having lunch the other day, to meet and get caught up on what we had been doing over the winter. She told me of her up and coming surgery to have her thyroid removed.

Her back teeth on both sides were giving her problems, so a week before her thyroid surgery, she was going to have a possible root canal on one or more teeth. I asked her, to please talk to her surgeon, before having the teeth work done, because the mouth is full of bacteria. I wanted her surgery to be successful. I had a tooth chart out in the car, so after lunch, she looked at the chart and compared her troubled teeth to the chart. Surprise! the teeth giving her the problems where the teeth representing the thyroid. That was a confirmation for her.

Mr. S. Writes "Linda, thank you for teaching me what stress is all about. I use to think tension headaches, knotted muscles, and sinus pain were a fact of life. I now know better. I haven't had a stress headache in weeks. My muscles feel much more relaxed, and my range of motion has increased noticeably. My wife says I no longer snore like a chainsaw. In addition, my sinus and allergy problems are the best they have been in the last ten years."

"Another aspect of your service, that I believe is truly important, is the way you educate your clients. I now understand the difference between survival and stress modes. I have put my body through both all these years on a constant basis. My stress is much more manageable."

About a year after 911, this traffic controller moved out a large metropolitan area with his family. He found that the stress in a large city airport was far too great on his health. Just think about the job he is doing. It's the duty of the traffic controller to get two planes in the same air space to land safely. He assists the pilot's to land safely. The pilots and crew get off the plane. The passengers all get off the plane, maybe not even aware of the emergency. They all go off and can relax, have fun or whatever they have planned to do.

However, the traffic controller may take five minutes, if he is lucky to relax and then get back to his high stress job that keeps him in survival mode. Even though he was not on those planes, his body feels as if he was. He may have several situations like this during that days shift. How can he get back to balancing his life in a happy way? He must learn the difference between stress and survival first. Happy to say he has!

Ms. C. She was a Magna Cum Laude graduate and pre-med student. Now in her late 50s, she is trying to live a holistic approach to life. She has had several surgeries and illnesses and spent many years in pain. Ms. C has fibromyalgia, chronic myofascial pain, degenerative disc disease, thyroid disease, osteoarthritis, calcific tendonitis, and multiple nerve impingements all, diagnosed by her doctors.

She wanted and desperately needed a better quality of life. Ms. C. had most of her dreams derailed, due to illness and pain. How does one unravel their body's pain when most often the pain is unbearable, both physically and emotionally? She has been to many doctors and specialists throughout the years, but most of time they only spend 10 to 15 minutes with her on each visit. Often her doctors classified her as one of their typical patients, prescribing either medication or surgery. She is not one of their typical patients. So, she has had to learn to listen to her own body. Whenever some pain comes up, she notes what has been going on in her life most recently. Then how did that incident make her feel?

She has learned how her body uniquely functions or does not function in relationship to her illness or pain. Ms. C. has changed her diet, and changed her posture. She uses a multiple of techniques to eliminate symptoms: gets low impact exercise, including water aerobics, salt baths, golf ball under her feet at least once a day, a cold water bottle behind her neck, and cold gel packs on her back, shoulders, hips and knees, as needed. She will not let pain last more than a few minutes before doing something to get it under control ASAP.

Fibromyalgia pain is nothing to reckon with, because that pain can create a domino effect. After the pain gets started, it is very difficult to get it to stop. Whenever she rides or drives in a car, she puts a cold water bottle behind her neck and sometimes when traveling long distance she will add a cold gel pack on her lower back, because she has had numerous whip lashes. She gets a massage a couple times a month and physical therapy when needed. Ms. C. has been using many of the techniques in this book for more than eight years now. She is into preventive medicine, self care and uses complementary medicine whenever possible.

Ms. B. Her life was full! Taking care of her Alzheimer husband at home and her mother-in-law was in an Alzheimer care facility. How did Ms. B. find time for herself? Believe it or not she would do some things for herself by taking her husband with her. Much like a mother would do with a per-school child. She came to one of my six week courses with him by her side and they never missed a class. She would bring him snacks so he could make it through the two hour class. I would keep my eye on him to make sure he did not get too agitated by what I was saying or doing.

He wanted to be a part of the class, if I was having the rest of the class do something active, he also, wanted to do it and sometimes it was more than he was capable of doing. He never spoke, so she and I would have to look for clues in him to prevent his outburst. Otherwise he could disrupt the class or worse yet she would have to leave.

When we got to the color class she asked how a color could help her husband. After finding out which color he responded to and how they worked for him she asked another question. "I have to take my mother-in-law out once a week to see her doctors or to get her hair done. She use to be pleasant to take out and I use to enjoy being with her. She has been my mother-in-law for almost 50 years and I still love very much. As she has gotten older and her Alzheimer's has gotten worse I find she has uncontrollable outburst more often and gets mad easy. I just can't seem to quiet her down, she seems to hate me all the time. I know she does not mean to act up or to hurt me but she does."

Seeing the cry for help in her eyes I calmly said, "Do you have any pink clothes in your closet?" She thought for a while and told us that she had a hot pink sweater and a soft pink blouse. I suggest that she wear the soft pink blouse when she took her mother-in-law out next and then come back to class and report how her day went. The next class she was back with a smile on her face, she was wearing a pink blouse and her husband was wearing a pink shirt. Why all this pink, we asked. She said with such joy in her voice; "wearing pink must have calmed my mother-in-law down, it was the best day we have had in a long time." She was so surprised with the pink she went out and bought a pink shirt for her husband, a couple more pink blouses for herself. Than with even a bigger smile on her face; she told us that she got a pink blouse for her mother-in-law and requested the care center put the pink blouse on her mother-in-law the days she was coming to be with her. Pink is everywhere around her now, on her, on her husband, on her mother-in-law and throughout her house. She has become the pink lady, carrying a great burden with Alzheimer, but a family full of love. As a smile on her face and a twinkle in her eye she cares for her love ones. She is an example and teacher on how LOVE + PINK = LIGHTENS UP YOUR HEART.

Ms. O. As the director of a Senior Center and so busy, she could only sit in on one of the six classes I was teaching. She had lost her husband two years earlier and had difficulty sleeping. She reported that she had not gotten a good night sleep since his death. I asked her, "What colors are you using in your bedroom?" I found out that it was purple and she was wearing purple that day. She also owned many things that were purple. I checked her and found purple was not a good color for her. I found that yellow was a calming color for her, suggesting that she might try wearing a yellow nightgown, to bed to see if she could sleep better. At the next class, she was so excited to tell the class of her experience using yellow. That first night, she did sleep better, but was not sure if it was the yellow she was wearing that helped her sleep. So she decided to wear yellow the next night. By the weekend, she got her grandson to paint her bedroom yellow and put up yellow drapes. She got yellow sheets and bedspread. Now, she is getting a good night sleep. I just reminded her to watch the full moon and new moon, if she isn't sleeping. She said she prayed to her husband, after he passed away, to help her sleep and now she prays to thank him for teaching her how to sleep without him.

Summary

In summary, self-renewal won't just happen to you. The best thing to do is to take time out each day for these life-balancing activities, even if it is fifteen or thirty minutes.

Well, this is the end of the book. Thank you for journeying with me and congratulations; you finished this book. Life is a progression of learning, trying and starting over and realizing there is more! I just want you to know that I truly believe in your future. Always remember that you were born with everything you need to succeed. Elvis Presley was told by one of his teachers that he was not good enough to be a singer and gave him a "C" in music. The power and the light are in you. Go out and show the world how happy and successful you can be at 100 years old. Be a mentor to others, let your true self shine! I wish you all the best and I leave you with a quote by Bob Moawad: You can't make footprints in the sand of time by sitting on your butt!

ants to leave butt prints in the sand of time!

Again, many thanks to everyone who has helped me get this book published. I could not have done it without all of you.

Also, a thank you goes out to the health care professionals practicing western and complementary medicine, who gave me the care I needed.

I want to thank my family and friends who stood beside me through the thick and thin in my journey.

I appreciate all of you expressing your kindness towards me. My healing depended upon your support. To all who encouraged me to write this book, I Thank you! To all of those whom I have worked with through the years, who have learned healing techniques and share them with others, I thank you!

If you want to know more on the up and coming classes in your area or become a trainer using these techniques you may contact: LindasJourney101@gmail.com.

References

"Take Five, the five elements, guide to health and harmony" by Pamela Ferguson

"Color Psychology and Color Therapy" by Vassily Kandinsky

"Colors and Numbers" by Louise L. Hay

"You Can Heal Your Life" by Louise L. Hay

"Going Deeper: Making the Invisible Visible" by Dr. Bernie Siegel, MD

"The Chopra Center Cookbook" by Deepak Chopra, MD, Dr David Simon, MD & Leanne Backer

"Change your Brain change your Life" by Daniel G. Amen, M.D.

"Inside Out" the movie by Pixar

"Babies" documentary movie by Universal and Focus Features

"The Skin, Tongue and Nails Speak" by Donna Burka Wild

"Good Grief" By Granger E. Westberg

"Passages in Care Giving" by Gail Sheehy

"The Power of Giving" by Azim Jamal and Harvey McKinnon

"The Power of Receiving" by Amanda Owens

"Outliers" by Malcolm Gladwell

"David and Goliath" by Malcolm Gladwell

"Ageless Body Timeless Mind" by Deepak Chopia

"How Successful People Think" by John C. Maxwell

"7 Principles of Fat Burning" by Eric Berg DC

"Super Foods" by David Wolfe

"Your Hands Can Heal You" by Master Co and Dr. Robins

"What Your Doctor May Not Tell You About Fibromyalgia" by R. Paul St. Amand and Claudia Craig Marek

Websites

www.mayoclinic.org   www.brainline.org

www.irleninstitute.com

About the Author

L inda Gifford has taught health classes in doctor offices, as well
as in the public sector. Including all ages of veteran's, people
with traumatic brain injuries and post traumatic stress disorder,
along with parents, children and caregivers. Her growing list of
students all started after 911 with firemen, policemen and traffic
controllers. Linda resides in Portland, Oregon.

CPSIA information can be obtained
at www.ICGtesting.com
Printed in the USA
FSOW01n0238070217
30473FS